THE BORN-AGAIN DIABETIC

THE HANDBOOK TO HELP YOU GET YOUR DIABETES IN CONTROL (AGAIN)

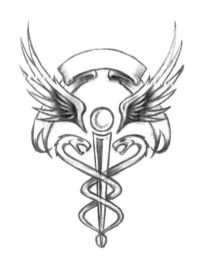

WILLIAM "LEE" DUBOIS

The Born-Again Diabetic
The handbook to help you get your diabetes in control (again)

Copyright © 2009 by William "Lee" Dubois

Published by
Red Blood Cell Books
P.O. Drawer A, Las Vegas, NM 87701
www.redbloodcellbooks.com

All rights reserved.

Cover concept and design by William "Lee" Dubois.
Title page and spine art: medical alert tattoo designed for
the author by Orlando Sedillo.

The information in this book is intended to help you make informed decisions about your health and the health of your loved ones. It is **not** intended to be a substitute for the treatment, advice, and care of your medical providers. While the author and publisher have endeavored to ensure that the information presented is accurate and up to date, they are not responsible for adverse effects or consequences sustained by any person using this book. Don't be a bone-head. Ask your doctor first.

ISBN 978-0-9822257-0-7

Printed in the United States of America

DEDICATION

This book is dedicated to my two children:

For my daughter **Morgan**, who by dying before she was born taught me the value of each and every human life…

And for my son **Rio** who lets me see the world afresh every day by the things his keen eyes see and by the questions he asks.

WILLIAM "LEE" DUBOIS

TABLE OF

Forward .... Page 1
Preface .... Page 5
Introduction .... Page 7

Section 1—Refresher: the Disease and the Risks .... Page 9

Chapter 1—So what the hell is diabetes, anyway? .... Page 11
Chapter 2—Complications from uncontrolled diabetes .... Page 23

Section 2—Fighting Back: the Power in Your Hands .... Page 29

Chapter 3—The Meter .... Page 31

Section 3—More about Blood, the Body, and Everything .... Page 61

Chapter 4—the A1C test and why it matters .... Page 65
Chapter 5—Food and blood .... Page 73
Chapter 6—Everything else and blood .... Page 81
Chapter 7—Why less is more .... Page 89
Chapter 8—Beyond blood .... Page 97

CONTENTS

Section 4—The Meds .... Page 111

    Chapter 9—Doctors, medications, and you .... Page 115
    Chapter 10—Oral diabetes medications .... Page 121
    Chapter 11—Injectable diabetes medications .... Page 133
    Chapter 12—Non-diabetes meds diabetics need .... Page 157

Section 5—The Real World .... Page 161

    Chapter 13—Sex, drugs, and rock & roll .... Page 163

Section 6—Ready, Set, Go! .... Page 181

    Chapter 14—Time to cross the finish line .... Page 183

Final thoughts .... Page 189

Acknowledgements .... Page 191

Resources .... Page 193

Glossary .... Page 195

Bibliography .... Page 203

Index .... Page 209

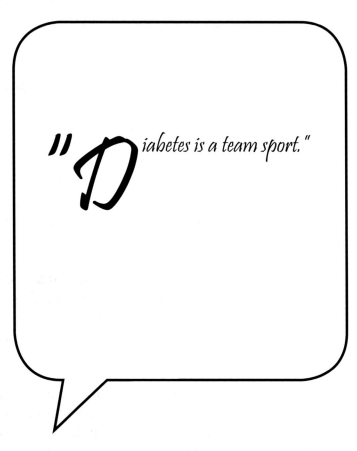

"Diabetes is a team sport."

Dr. Kathleen Colleran, Endocrinologist
...and author of our forward

Forward by Kathleen Colleran, MD

*D*on't let the title of this book mislead you. Contrary to what you might think at first glance, "The Born-Again Diabetic" has little if anything to do with religion, and everything to do with day-to-day reality.

Think of this book as the ultimate diabetes travel guide. After reading it, you will understand everything the doctors, nurses, and educators told you—and more importantly, everything they didn't tell you that may be more pertinent for your journey as a diabetic.

Lee Dubois, the author of this book, uses wit, personal experience, and professional expertise to accurately describe the nuts and bolts of living successfully with diabetes. He does this with both humor and colorful language, but also with dead-on accuracy.

*I first met Mr. Dubois in 2006 at Diabetes Day at the New Mexico State Capitol, an annual event to recognize diabetes programs throughout our state. Mr. Dubois' clinic had a table next to my partner, New Mexico Takes on Diabetes, and me. I was promoting the **E**xtension for **C**ommunity **H**ealth **O**utcomes for diabetes, the ECHO diabetes project, a program* *to train providers to attain better outcomes for diabetes via telemedicine.*

Being in close proximity to Dubois' table and its boisterous presence, it was clear that Mr. Dubois was at ease and thoroughly enjoyed engaging and educating people about diabetes. In fact, I falsely assumed he was a doctor at the clinic because his demeanor, rapport and more specifically his knowledge, were riveting.

After he corrected me as to his title, I was humbled, but even more impressed. Since then we have become comfortable colleagues. We readily share resources, patient experiences, and knowledge.

Mr. Dubois is a poster child for my philosophy that it's not the alphabet soup following your name (MD, MPA, CDE, RD, XYZ, etc.) that matters; rather it's the content of the bowl that matters. More important than titles is what you know, what you can learn, and what you realize you do not know. I've told him more than once that it is your name that matters, not what follows it.

Mr. Dubois has no alphabet soup after his name. In fact, having on first meeting mistaken him for a doctor, imagine my shock when I discovered that he was originally a high school dropout. His education in diabetes care comes from an unquenchable thirst for knowledge, and from personal experience.

Attempting to defy statistics, Mr. Dubois developed Type-1 Diabetes in his forties. Sometimes I actually wonder if he did it on purpose, as his sole mission outside of family seems to be to help patients, families, medical providers, communities, and society overcome the myths and stigma that surround diabetes. This book is not about religion, but I think diabetes is almost a religion to him.

He has poured his heart and soul and brain into improving diabetes care for over 400 people with diabetes in his community. And that is just direct care. Like ripples from a stone thrown in a pond, his efforts help patients he has never met. I think this book will make an even bigger splash.

Through diligence, he has gained the respect of the providers in his community and nearby communities. In addition to his full-time work at the clinic, Mr. Dubois is a member of the steering committee of the New Mexico Diabetes Advisory Council, the tool kit work group of New Mexico Takes on Diabetes, and sits on the state board of the New Mexico Branch of the American Diabetes Association. He is also a champion for the Project ECHO diabetes program, where we work "together," via video link, once every week.

As Mr. Dubois so aptly states, remember you did not choose diabetes, it chose you. So live long and prosper... and enjoy the book, and most importantly, the journey.

About Dr. Colleran

Physician, teacher, scientist, Kathleen Colleran, MD, has a dazzling resume. Starting at the University of Wisconsin, first earning her BS in Molecular Biology and then earning her MD, she moved to the Scholar's Program at the School of Medicine at the University of New Mexico in 1999, where she is now Associate Professor of Medicine. Dr. Colleran also serves as Medical Director of the Clinical Trials Center, Medical Director of the Cardiovascular Risk Reduction Clinic, and Program Director of the Endocrinology and Metabolism Fellowship.

Dr. Colleran is certified by the American Board of Internal Medicine and the American Board of Endocrinology and Metabolism and has received numerous professional recognitions and honors. She is in constant demand as a lecturer and has published endless articles and abstracts in the scholarly press, including such publications as The New England Journal of Medicine and Diabetes Care.

She is a member of the American Diabetes Association, the Endocrine Society, and the American College of Physicians. For years, she served as camp physician for the American Diabetes Association's Diabetes Camp. She currently serves as Western Region President of the American Federation for Medical Research. She gives half a day a week to outpatient Endocrine Clinics and six weeks of each year she works in inpatient general medicine wards. She has sat on endless committees, mentored dozens of medical students, and of course—last but not least—given her all for the ECHO Telemedicine program, sharing her knowledge and expertise with primary care providers statewide.

Preface

A debate rages within our "tribe." Are we *Diabetics* or are we *Persons with Diabetes*? This is no small semantic tussle. For many patients, being defined by their medical condition is insulting, demoralizing, and may lead to a self-fulfilling prophecy of defeat.

The concept behind *Person with Diabetes*, often abbreviated PWD, is that you are a person first and foremost, who just happens to have a condition. I'm sorry. I'm not a member of the PWD camp.

First, why use three words instead of one? Especially when you write about diabetes a lot, it can get tedious saying *Person with Diabetes* every time you need to.

Second, we generally don't say Person with Asthma, Person with Cancer, Person with the Flu. While I do respect the concept and I applaud anything that makes a person feel better, I confess that I find it a bit silly.

Third, and most importantly, I am proud to be *Diabetic*. I wear my alert jewelry openly. I talk about diabetes at every opportunity. I even have a medical alert tattoo on my wrist that says "Diabetic," not Person with Diabetes.

The general public has a lot to learn about diabetes. As a *Diabetic* or as a *Person with Diabetes*, we are ambassadors. Be Diabetic or be PWD, but be proud. Don't waste your breath explaining to the lay public why you are a *Person with Diabetes*, not a *Diabetic*. Instead, use your breath to educate on the real issues.

In this book, both because of my beliefs and because of my desire to keep my poor little fingers from overworking, I will refer to *us* as diabetics.

If you are a PWD please take no insult and know that I love you just the same.

Lee

Introduction
...the day you were dx'd

Most people remember very little about the day they were diagnosed, beyond their doctor telling them "you have diabetes." Everything that was said after that disappears into an odd fog, like the "wah-wha-wah-wha" of adult voices in *Peanuts* TV specials.

Probably your doctor told you a great deal. But all you heard was your inner voice: *Diabetes? I can't possibly have diabetes!*

Maybe you had the misfortune to meet with a nurse or diabetes educator on that first day. Or worse yet, a dietitian. If so, it was too early, and you were bombarded with more information than you could possibly absorb.

You were probably given pamphlets that were either so dumbed down you couldn't learn a thing, or were so biased toward a particular medication that it made you ill.

You were probably given a blood glucose meter. Maybe you were taught how to use it, maybe you weren't. Maybe you were but that voice in your head saying *Diabetes? I can't possibly have diabetes!* was so loud you couldn't hear the instructions.

If you went online when you got home, you probably scared the hell out of yourself.

You probably just went to bed that first day, hoping you'd wake up and it would all be a bad dream. Well, it was a bad dream—but you were awake and this was your new life.

Of course you pulled yourself together. You began to learn what you needed to know. You learned how to test your blood sugar, how to take your medications, what food and drink your body liked and what it did not. You probably even started to exercise. You took control because you were scared.

Then time passed. Little by little you began to slip back into your old comfort zone, the way you had always lived your life. Bit by bit, like a thief in the night, your diabetes began to creep up on you. It is an insidious disease. It is *chronic*: meaning permanent. It never goes away. It is *progressive*: meaning that every day you live it gets a little worse. And if that were not enough, your body adapts to your medications. Little by little they lose their effectiveness. And to top it all off, the symptoms of diabetes damage don't really show up until it is too late. Once you feel it, the damage is done.

Today you woke up and realized you'd lost control.

It is time. You are ready. You are ready to take back your diabetes. Roll up your sleeves and let's get to work together! You are **the born again diabetic**, and this book will remind you of the things you forgot, update you on the things that have changed, and teach you the things you never learned.

Section 1—Refresher: the Disease and the Risks

Chapter 1—So what the hell is diabetes anyway?..........................Page 11

This chapter covers the kinds of diabetes and the causes of diabetes. Together, we'll talk about Type-1, Type-1.5, Type-2, and Type-3, plus pre-diabetes and gestational diabetes. The chapter explains how each kind happens, who gets each kind, and how the various kinds of diabetes differ from each other and what they have in common. We'll also cover some interesting trivia. This chapter puts you into context in our larger "tribe."

> Type-1 Diabetes..Page 11
> Type-1.5 Diabetes... Page 14
> Type-2 Diabetes .... Page 15
> Hey, what about pre-diabetes?.. Page 19
> Gestational Diabetes.. Page 20
> Type-3 Diabetes... Page 21

Chapter 2—Complications from uncontrolled diabetes......................Page 23

This chapter walks you through all the scary things that can happen to you if you let your diabetes get the upper hand. It covers damage to your blood vessels, eyes, kidneys, nerves, and heart. I'll tell you how high blood sugar can cause all of this damage; and how many people it happens to. We'll also talk about amputations. And death.

> **DI•A•BE'•TES** *(NOUN)*
>
> A disease associated with inadequate production of insulin by the pancreas... untreated, the disease is commonly fatal.

Funk & Wagnalls New Practical Dictionary
1954 *(relax, a lot has changed since then)*

Chapter 1—So what the hell is diabetes, anyway?

In a nutshell, diabetes is a variety of conditions that make it hard for your body to deal with sugar. There are four types of diabetes. In the medical world we define them as:

Type-1
Type-1.5
Type-2
And Gestational Diabetes

For what it is worth, we'll also talk about Type-3s. So I guess there are five types; except for the fact 2s and GDs can be lumped together as we'll soon see, as can 1s and 1.5s.

Type-1 Diabetes

I'm a T-1 myself. We're a rare breed, making up only about 5% of the diabetes population. T-1 used to be called "Juvenile Diabetes" because it often struck early in life. We've kicked that term to the curb 'cause we're now seeing older folks develop this version of diabetes.

T-1 is an autoimmune disorder. The body's immune system attacks and kills off the insulin-producing beta cells in the *pancreas* (the small ugly-looking organ that hides behind your stomach and causes so much trouble for all us D-folk). What does that mean in plain English? Insulin is a hormone that allows sugar to be used by the body. Every cell in your body—from a brain cell, to a coronary artery cell, to a skin cell in your little toe—eats a type of sugar called *glucose*. That's how the cells live. The entire job of your digestive system is to convert anything that goes into your mouth into glucose. From Twinkies to T-bones, all that you eat becomes glucose.

The analogy that is often used is to picture each cell in your body as having a locked door. Insulin is the key that unlocks the door and lets the glucose in. I absolutely *hate* this analogy, but I've yet to come up with anything better on my own.

So, without any insulin, there is no way for glucose—the fuel for the entire body—to get into the cells. Prior to 1922, all Type-1 diabetics died. Period. Type-1 was an always-fatal disease until two saints by the names of Best and Banting worked out what insulin is, how to capture it, refine it, and use it as a medicine.

All Type-1s take insulin. We need it with every bite of food we eat, and we need it at night while we sleep. Pills will not work for us. We must take insulin. T-1 is more common in populations of European descent, but can show up in any racial or ethnic group.

How does Type-1 happen? Good frickin' question, and some of the brightest minds in medical science have struggled with this question for decades. Bottom line: no one really knows. The best and most popular guess is that T-1 results from a combination of a genetic predisposition and an "unknown" trigger. What that means is that some peoples' bodies are designed in such a way that, given the right circumstances, our immune systems freak out and attack the home team.

Of course, if it were really that simple, we'd expect T-1 to cluster in family groups. This, for the most part, is not the case. Most T-1s rarely meet a fellow patient in the wild. I'm the only one in my family even out to fourth cousins three times removed. There are cases of sibs having T-1; or of it appearing over several generations, but that is the exception rather than the rule. Maybe we've only been able to live long enough to reproduce for so few generations that the genetic nature of the disease is only beginning to show up. Or maybe not.

As to the trigger. Historically T-1 hit around puberty, but now we see two new trends—juvenile diagnosis is happening at progressively younger ages and full-grown adults are developing T-1 as well.

Why? One thought is that if you are genetically predisposed you'll get T-1 Diabetes whenever you encounter the "trigger," whatever the Sam Hill the trigger actually is. Maybe a virus, think some. Maybe environmental pollution. Maybe the moon is in Leo, the wind is from the west, the barometric pressure is dropping….

The only reason the cause matters, is that to cure T-1 Diabetes, we really need to understand it. For decades researchers have thought they were on the brink of a cure, only to be repulsed time and time again. In the 1970's parents were told it really didn't matter how good or bad the blood sugar control of their children was because T-1 would be cured in a few years. Many of those patients have died horrible deaths.

If you are T-1 or the parent of a T-1, heed my advice: hope for a cure; but live every day as if there will never be one.

Type-1.5 Diabetes

Well, like Big Foot and the Loch Ness Monster, not everyone in medicine agrees that T-1.5 even exists at all. The term was first coined when adults started developing T-1; and at the time it was generally accepted that *that* was not supposed to happen. Type-1.5 diabetes is also called LADA, which stands for Latent Autoimmune Diabetes in Adults. Really, there is not much difference between 1.5 and T-1.

However, 1.5 does hit later, after age 30, and the body's production of insulin drops off more gradually than it typically does with younger T-1s, but that does not necessarily mean it is a different disorder. One Endocrinologist (Latin for Diabetes and Thyroid doctor) I know classified 1.5 as those who are not quite T-1s; they still had some insulin production, but could not survive without some supplemental insulin shots.

I generally lump 1.5's in with T-1s and can feel justified in doing so 'cause I myself could be classified as a T-1.5. I developed my diabetes at age 40. At the time, as I was an overweight middle-aged white guy, my primary care physician assumed I had Type-2 diabetes and put me on some pills, whereupon I got really sick. Referred for an emergency Endo visit (which took 6 weeks to get) I was declared to be a Type 1.5, was given various insulins, and began a new life. At the next visit a month or two later, I was told that the lab tests showed my body was not producing a single drop of insulin.

"Congratulations," my Endo told me, "you've been promoted to a Type-1."

Type-2 Diabetes

Type-2 is by far the most common kind of diabetes in the world, and it is growing at near epidemic rates. Many experts argue that it is already an epidemic. Recent data from the American Diabetes Association (guaranteed to be out of date by the time you read this) estimates that 8% of the population of the United States has been formally diagnosed with diabetes, and that the best guess is that a much larger number are walking around unaware they have it. If you were given the "bad news" today, you'd be only one of over 4,000 Americans who were having the same bad day. Mind boggling.

T-2 is a horse of a different color from T-1 or T-1.5. It starts as a disease of *insulin resistance*. So what is insulin resistance, you ask? OK, let's go back to our lousy (but best option) analogy from the discussion of Type-1. If you skipped over that 'cause you're a Type-2 and thought reading about T-1s didn't matter, you need to go back and read that section before going on.

So here goes the little insulin hormone molecule on its merry way up to the cell to unlock the door to let the sugar in so the cell can eat. Standing on the doorstep of the cell, the insulin reaches into its pocket and is horrified to find that it brought the car keys, not the house keys. The insulin is there, but it can't unlock the door.

Meanwhile, the cell is getting hungrier and hungrier. It's on the phone to the pancreas: "Hey, I ordered a pizza up here over an hour ago and the driver still hasn't shown up." The pancreas, not knowing what's going on, sends more insulin molecules into the body. Most of them with the car keys. Type-2's bodies are flooded with insulin, at least for a few years.

Enough insulin leaves with the house keys that the body does not starve, but there are not enough of the house-key-carrying insulin molecules to keep the blood sugar at healthy levels. The blood sugar levels creep up a little at a time over months or years. It is such a slow onset that most patients don't even feel it happening.

Yeah, they don't have as much energy as they used to. Yeah, they pee a lot, but they're drinking a lot of water lately. Yeah, they think, my vision isn't what it used to be, I probably need new glasses. I'll take care of that soon.

All symptoms of high blood sugar.

Meanwhile, like any machine that is overworked and gets no rest, the pancreas eventually breaks down. Overworked, it can no longer make enough of the magic hormone and the T-2 must start taking insulin shots like his T-1 cousins; and a heck of a lot more of it as the insulin-dependent T-2 still suffers from the original insulin resistance plus the newly developed lack of insulin production. Most T-2s who live long enough will take insulin. It doesn't mean they are "bad" or sicker. It is just the way it is. So have they been "promoted" to Type-1s? Technically, no. Even though the treatment may be the same, the root causes are different.

T-1 is a defect in the immune system. Insulin-dependant T-2 is a case of an overworked pancreas that can no longer keep up with the body's needs. Same treatment, but horses of different colors. Once a T-1, always a T-1. Once a T-2, always a T-2.

So what causes this insulin resistance in the first place? Genetics play a key role. We see Type-2 diabetes cluster strongly in families. Mother, father, sibs, grandparents, aunts and uncles, cousins. Type-2 is a family affair. Well, usually. Every once in a while I get an abused-feeling patient who is the first person in the family tree to get diabetes. It is important to remember that every human is the joining of two family trees. Your father's side maybe didn't have it. Your mother's side maybe didn't have it. But you do. Well, something new happened when merging your Mom's DNA and your Dad's DNA. All diabetes had to start somewhere, right? But now that you have it, your children are at extraordinarily high risk. That's just the way it is.

This brings us back to triggers. In the case of T-2 there are two triggers and we know what they are: age and weight. If you are predisposed to T-2, you will get it if you get old enough or fat enough. On the other hand, there are lots of really fat people who don't have diabetes. They were not genetically predisposed. Simply being fat, even morbidly so, is not enough by itself to cause diabetes. If it were, our diabetes rates in the United States would be closer to 65%.

A lot of folks think they gave themselves diabetes by eating too many Snickers bars. That's mostly not true. I've actually had patients break down and cry when they realized it wasn't "their fault." They'd been carrying around a huge load of guilt, but just eating sugar does not give you diabetes. Your body has to be set up for it. It's the weight that you gain from eating Snickers bars that triggers the insulin resistance that causes the diabetes. Not the actual sugar. The shin bone's connected to the knee bone, the knee bone's connected to the thigh bone.... *Of course in the medical world we say the tibia connects to the patella, the patella connects to the femur....*

I digress. There is a society-wide feeling that being "fat" is the cause of diabetes, so you brought it on yourself. A lot of T-1s who encounter this kind of mindless prejudice get hot under the collar, feeling that they did nothing to bring this on themselves. This is true, but it is also true that the overweight T-2s have done nothing to bring diabetes on themselves either. Obesity is a social disease. We humans are products of the environments we live in, even if we've created those very environments ourselves. Even if those environments are hostile and unhealthy.

Americans are FAT. I kid you not. And getting fatter every year. It is a combination of diet, changes in activity patterns, and a whole lot of other things. Too much to cover right here, but I'll talk more about it later.

For what it's worth, being fat isn't as simple as it sounds. Once the body has shifted into a fat-storing mode it's difficult to break back out of. Certain elements of T-2 diabetes make it doubly difficult to lose weight. In fact, the condition makes it easier to gain weight, and the more weight you gain the worse the condition and the worse the condition the more weight and so on.... It is a vicious cycle that is damn hard to break.

T-2 used to hit at middle age, as that is when most of us start packing on the pounds. Now that we have a national obesity crisis at all age levels we are seeing many cases of full-blown T-2 in children as young as nine years old, and sometimes even younger.

Developing T-2 this young will shave 20 years off their lives, as early onset requires them to live with T-2 diabetes far longer than their bodies can handle. Medically, we say these children will predecease their parents. In plain English, they will die before their parents do.

People whose skin has an interesting tint are more likely to have T-2 than people who have pale skin. Hispanics and African-Americans are much more likely to develop T-2 than their paler neighbors, as are folks of Asian descent. In some Native American tribes diabetes is the rule, rather than the exception. But don't kid yourself if you are white. Plenty of white people have T-2 diabetes.

Hey, what about pre-diabetes?

So your doctor told you that you had pre-diabetes, or borderline diabetes? Sorry, I'm here to tell you that you can't be a little bit pregnant.

Technically, we define diabetes as a certain absolute blood sugar number. One point over and you are a member of our club—we'll mail you a T-shirt and a blood glucose monitor while supplies last. One point under and you aren't diabetic.

But your blood sugar is waaaaaay higher than a "normal" person's yet not high enough to be diabetic; so what the Sam Hill do we do with you? Most doctors will tell you that you have pre-diabetes, which sounds so harmless you probably won't do diddly squat about it. There actually isn't even a medical diagnosis, what we call an ICD-9 code, for pre-diabetes. The closest I've been able to find is "abnormal blood glucose not otherwise classified."

I don't believe in pre-diabetes. If you fall into this range you are a T-2 diabetic that does not need medication yet; and it is better to accept that fact.

Gestational Diabetes

If you are a man this won't happen to you. Gestational diabetes is often viewed as a "temporary" diabetes that strikes some pregnant women. Actually it'll hit more than 4% of pregnant women—over 135,000 American women last year—and the rate is rising.

But I'm here to share a secret. It really isn't some mysterious temporary ailment that will go away. We should rename it. It should be called *Preview Diabetes*.

Gestational diabetes is your crystal ball. Your look into the future. If you had GD, I'll put money on the fact that once you are old enough or heavy enough, you'll get T-2. The distilled fact of the matter is that a pregnancy is so hard on a woman's body that it temporarily fast-forwards her age about 10 years.

So we've got an increase in "age" and an increase in weight and *boom*: diabetes shows up. After giving birth it goes away in most cases. *But it isn't really gone.* It is lurking under the surface like a hungry shark waiting for her to get old enough or fat enough…

Type-3 Diabetes

Type-3 diabetics aren't actually diabetics at all. Well, not in most cases, anyway. As far as I know, the term was coined by the folks at dLife. dLife is an empire of sorts that involves web sites, a TV show, multimedia, books, and more. They dreamed up the tag of T-3 for the family members of any of the other types of diabetics. It is a way of symbolizing that diabetes doesn't just affect the patient; it affects the patient's entire family.

So Type-3s are commonly spouses, but can be parents, children, or sibs of diabetics.

I loved the term as soon as I heard it. We even have Type-3 support and education groups at my clinic now. In our communities the term is as well known as Type-2 Diabetes is. It's not uncommon for someone I've never seen before to poke their head into my office and without preamble say, "I'm a Type-3 Diabetic and I have a question about my (husband-wife-daughter-son-uncle-aunt's) blood sugar."

If you love a Type-1, Type-1.5, Type-2, or a woman with gestational diabetes, you are a Type-3 diabetic.

> "The words 'diabetic' and 'diabolic' occur so closely together in the dictionary, there must be some way to make a play on words about that."

Kathy Dubois Reed, Type-3 Diabetic
Playwright, & the Author's Sister

Chapter 2—Complications from uncontrolled diabetes

Complications. Sounds harmless. Gosh, these Lego instructions are complicated. Using the new software at work is complicated. Programming the frickin' VCR is complicated.

No big deal, just complicated. Nothing that can't be solved with a little brain work, right?

Wrong. Complications from diabetes are devastating, often permanent, side effects of out-of-control diabetes that can kill you. I'm not smart enough to come up with a chilling enough word to replace *complications*, but we definitely need something better. If you develop complications, your life will be more than complicated. It will be awful.

Here's the deal, straight talk, no feel-good bullshit: high levels of blood sugar can and will destroy every part of your body.

Actually, for what it is worth, diabetes in itself is perfectly harmless. It doesn't and can't hurt you in any way. All diabetes does is make it hard for your body to deal with metabolizing sugar.

Here is a fun little science experiment. Go buy some fresh strawberries and a half pound of sugar. Put a dozen or so of the berries in a bowl and pour some sugar over them. Add a little water for the heck of it and throw them in the fridge. Wait 24-to-48 hours.

What happened?

The strawberries turned into mush, didn't they? Why? Because that's what sugar does. That's what sugar in your blood can do to your internal organs. It will break them down, turn them into mush too.

Quick biology lesson: you remember the red blood cell, right? Looks like a Martian flying saucer? Red blood cells are the FedEx trucks of your body, moving oxygen from the lungs to the cells and carrying out the trash. Well, OK, I guess I've never actually seen the FedEx guy taking out the trash, but….

Your blood travels through miles and miles and miles of tubing inside your body: the circulatory system. To be exact, if you took the average human's circulatory system and stretched it out you'd have 60,000 miles of highway for your blood cells to travel on…well, in. Everyone's heard of the big players. Aorta. Jugular. Let me introduce you to the pawn on the chessboard. The capillary. Smallest part of this network. Hey, every cell needs food and oxygen, right? So red blood cells need a way to get to all the trillions of cells that make up *you*. At the far end of your own personal universe live the *distal capillaries*. They are the smallest of the small, and logically enough are at the far ends of your body…your toes and fingertips.

There are two, well, four actually, other places where we find lots, and lots, and lots of capillaries. More on that in a minute.

Some of these capillaries are soooo small that they are actually smaller in diameter than the cells that pump through them. Remember our little red Martian flying saucers? Well, now you need to think of them as pancakes. Under normal circumstances they are flexible. They can hunch their little shoulders and wriggle through the capillary.

Unless they are encrusted in sugar. Then the pancakes become Frisbees.

I'll leave it to your imagination as to what happens when a rigid object forces itself through a slightly too small soft-tissue space. Uh huh. I think you got the visual I wanted you to have.

I mentioned that there are a couple of places in the body besides the distal capillaries where the circulatory system features lots of small tubes. One, er, two, are your eyes. Yep, the back of your retina…basically the eyeball. If a bunch of capillaries rupture in the back of the eyeball you will go blind. Irreversibly blind. Diabetic eye trouble is called *retinopathy*.

Diabetics suffer 20,000 cases of blindness per year.

And if that doesn't suck enough, let's talk about your kidneys. If you see one in a jar, it doesn't look like much. A kidney-bean shaped dark red-brown organ. Looks dense. Don't judge this filter by its cover. It is actually a huge mass of capillaries. One of the most amazing, beautiful, and scary things I've ever seen was at one of the traveling Body Worlds exhibits. Body Worlds took real human cadavers (dead folks) and preserved them in unique ways, often injecting them with various silicones and then displaying the bodies in artistic ways. It's an amazing, educational and artistic journey inside of *us*. Highly recommended.

At Body Worlds I saw a kidney. The capillaries had been filled up with silicone and the tissue dissolved away to reveal the inner structure.

Wow! How to describe.... A three dimensional spider web? An organic circuit board? A tangle of roots below the sod of a fine Kentucky bluegrass? An insane California freeway seen from the space shuttle? All of these fall short of describing the incredibly complex, beautiful tangle of filtering capillaries. Dense, delicate, wonderful—and easily trashed by high sugar.

When the kidneys start to fail from high blood sugar, the first thing that slips through is *microalbumin*; which are little tiny protein molecules. We can test your urine to see if microalbumin is spilling through the kidneys. That is the early warning sign. There is still time to change. Once full-sized proteins show up in the urine the possibility of dialysis is very, very, very real. Diabetic kidney trouble is called *nephropathy*.

Diabetics suffer more than 44,000 cases of kidney failure per year, and 44% percent of all patients on dialysis are diabetic. In fact, diabetes is the single leading cause of kidney failure. I worked for a time in an Intensive Care Unit (ICU) at a large regional medical center. An alarming number of our "guests" were out-of-control diabetics in *End Stage Renal Failure*—in plain English, kidney failure. The portable dialysis machine went from one ICU bay to the next, to the next, to the next…all day long.

It was too much for me. I got the hell out of there and found a job that lets me try to intervene earlier. *It is now my goal to really hurt the bottom line of the ICU.*

65% of diabetics also suffer from *neuropathy*—nerve damage caused by high blood sugars. It comes in two flavors. In one version it causes terrible pain in the feet and hands, *all the time*. Right out of Dante. In the other version you don't feel anything in your feet, which can lead to our next complication:

Diabetics suffer 84,000 "non-traumatic" amputations per year. I guarantee you that any amputation is traumatic. What we are saying here is that these were medically necessary amputations rather than cases of some poor sod running over his foot with the lawn mower. Sometimes a diabetic loses a toe. Or two or three. Sometimes a foot to the ankle. Or a leg to the knee. Or a leg to the hip. We take as little as we can. People who lose toes often are back again to lose more. We kill them a slice at a time. Diabetic amputations happen because as neuropathy develops, you can't feel your feet. If you step on a tack or a nail or get a splinter, you don't feel it. You have no awareness it is there. If your blood sugar is high, it impairs your body's ability to heal. A minor injury becomes an infected one, the infection becomes an abscess, the abscess becomes gangrene, and the gangrene must be cut off. At that point the affected flesh is dead.

And speaking of dead:

Diabetics suffer 135,000 fatal heart attacks per year.

Well, now that I've scared the crap out of you, I want you to know that none, repeat, *none* of these statistics needs to exist at all. Remember, diabetes is harmless. It is the sugar that kills and maims. Keep your blood sugar in control and you'll be surrounded by laughing great-grandchildren with your eyes sharp, your kidneys filtering all the blood in your body every 30 minutes, and all your toes in your fuzzy slippers.

That is what this book is all about: *to remind you of the things you forgot, update you on the things that have changed, and teach you the things you never learned.* Come on, let's go get healthy again!

Section 2—Fighting Back: the Power in Your Hands

Chapter 3—The meter....................Page 31

This chapter covers the Power and Purpose of meters; those humble little boxes for checking your blood sugar that can make or break your diabetes control. We'll talk about how they work and how to use them; and how often you should use yours. It covers what the numbers mean and what to do with those numbers. We're also going to touch on high and low blood sugar, some important tips, and how to carry your meter. The chapter wraps up by reviewing key numbers and key management strategies and then we'll peek into the future-that-is-now by telling you all about Continuous Glucose Monitors.

How does a meter work?	Page 33
Using the meter in the "trenches"	Page 39
How often should I check my blood sugar?	Page 40
The numbers and what they mean	Page 43
How low can you go?	Page 44
How high can you get?	Page 47
Two important things you need to know about your meter	Page 48
Where does your meter live?	Page 52
Checkmate—the meter as the best weapon to master your diabetes	Page 53
Summary—the 10 Commandments of Meters	Page 54
Your target numbers are:	Page 55
Beyond meters	Page 55

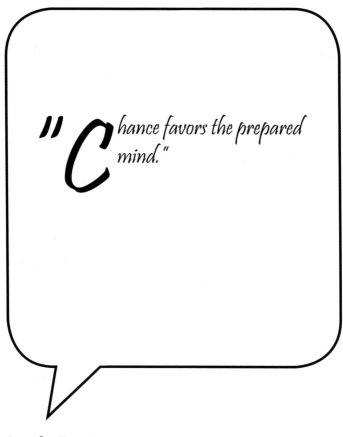

"*Chance favors the prepared mind.*"

Louis Pasteur
19th-Century Scientist

Chapter 3—The meter

The fundamental, indispensable tool for controlling diabetes has only been around since 1980 or so. Yep, the humble blood glucose meter. As the meter is the single most important self-management tool in your arsenal, we're going to devote quite a bit of time to it in this chapter. Trust me, your meter is your best friend.

You have in the palm of your hand the ability to diagnostically assess your health, day or night, every day of the week. You get results in seconds and it costs you only $1 at the most. What could be better? Just ask any woman waiting for the results of her mammogram.

Diabetes is actually a wonderful disease to have. No really, hear me out. What other condition can be *self-managed?* Yeah, you have a doctor, a diabetes educator, maybe a dietitian, maybe an Endo.

Hopefully, you have a lot of help, but it is *your* diabetes. *You* are in the driver's seat. You are in-control or out-of-control. It is your choice.

Your meter is a tool that lets you look inside your body. You have been given the ultimate crystal ball. You can even do your own "one-rat" clinical research. Want to know how the super-sized French fries at McDonalds treat your blood sugar? *Test, don't guess.*

Take a reading before eating. Eat. Test again at 30 minutes, an hour, two hours, three hours. Think about the results. Let the results guide you.

Maybe you love fries but your poor diabetic body does not. Maybe the super-size experiment ended badly, but maybe you can tolerate a small bag. Use your tools and your brain to take control of your diabetes.

The meter, sometimes called a glucometer or blood glucose meter or blood testing meter or….*where was I?* Oh yes, the meter really is a miracle product. Before meters the only way to test your blood sugar was to pee on a strip and go through a lengthy ritual involving boiling water and color comparison charts. It was slow, tedious, inaccurate and in any case only told you where your blood sugar was hours before.

Your meter is the first line of defense against complications. Used wisely it can warn you of trouble ahead, both short and long term. It tells you what foods your body loves and what foods your body hates. It can warn you about dangerously high or dangerously low blood sugar levels. It can tell you if your medications are working for you. It alerts you when your diabetes goes to the next level. And it will. It's progressive, remember?

Pathetically, most D-folk have no idea how to really get the most out of their meters. That changes today!

There are now dozens of meters to choose from in a variety of shapes, sizes and colors. On top of my little insulin fridge at the clinic I have a sample of every meter we have in-house. There are 21 of them. People often ask, "Why do you have so many cell phones?" My answer: *I gotta stay in touch with my diabetes.*

The meters sport a dazzling array of features that you'll never use. What is the very best meter on the market? The one you can get strips for.

There are no generic meters. Nor are there generic strips, the disposable thin plastic lab-in-a-tab that allows the meter to read your blood sugar. Strips cost a dollar each over the counter, and few diabetics are rich enough to pay for the number they really need. Insurance companies do not want to pay for as many strips as you need, nor is there patient assistance for test strips.

I confess: I'm a test-strip whore. I'll use any kind I can get my mitts on. We get a limited number of samples at the clinic as new models are introduced. I try them all. Some I like better than others, but in the end a strip is just a strip, and a meter is just a meter.

How does a meter work?

Well, as far as I can tell, meters are magic. To be honest, I've read dozens of technical articles on the electro-bio-chemistry of the various meter systems, but I still can't honestly say I really understand how the damn things work. You just have to take it on faith. After all, you drive your car just fine without really understanding everything that happens under the hood, right? You use your computer just fine without understanding the wiring, chips, and assorted mysteries, right?

All meter systems have three separate components. First is the meter itself. Usually smaller than a cell phone, it is the brains of the system. You should get a new one every three years; they tend to get funky when they get old. And for God's sake never pay for one. I'm amazed that meters are even offered for sale at all. Look, all the meter companies want you to be their slave. To use their strips you must own their meter. There is no money to be made selling meters; but boy, is there ever money to be made selling strips. Do the math yourself. If we take the 17.9 million *diagnosed* U.S. diabetics at last count, and if they all tested an average of only three times a day (*not enough! But more on that later…*), and the strips are a dollar each, that makes test strips a *nineteen billion one hundred seventeen million two hundred thousand dollar* per year market in the United States alone. Never mind the rest of the world where the exportation of the fast food lifestyle has triggered a global obesity epidemic that is waking up dormant T-2 genes in populations that don't even know what the word means.

Most doctors' offices, hospitals, and diabetes educators have closets full of meters. Failing that, many meter companies host health fairs where they give them out. Sometimes your insurance company will send you one free. As a side note, one of the insane things about many insurance companies is that they understand, on one level, that if you test often and take care of yourself, you will cost them a lot less in the long run; yet on the other hand, they are greedy profit-grubbing bastards who'd sell their own mothers into slavery to make fifty cents today. That's why they'll give you a free meter, but won't pay for enough strips to run it right. *Oh, my. Maybe I should have a drink and calm down.*

As a last resort, Google the meter company, call them up and tell them you'd love to use their product, their strips would be covered by your insurance, but you can't seem to find a meter anywhere, and then just sit back and wait for the UPS truck.

The next component of the system is test strips. They are thin flexible plastic matchsticks between half an inch and an inch long; usually an eighth inch or so wide. They are actually quite a bit more complex than they appear; sandwiched between the plastic top and bottom is quite a bit of science. The strips are designed to wick in a small blood sample for analysis by the meter. They are disposable one-shot wonders. Usually they come in vials reminiscent of the little plastic tubs 35mm film used to come in. It is *important* that you keep the strips in the little tub and keep the cotton-pickin' lid shut except to get a strip out. This is important because the vial is more than packaging. It contains a lining that keeps the strips dry and preserved. As one of our patients discovered, if you just throw them into a zip-lock bag for convenience, the strips will get funky on you and give you crazy readings.

The vials vary in size. Some are very easy to get a single strip out of but are a bigger pain in the ass to carry around with you, and others are petite but usually result in all the strips ending up on the floor a couple of times per month.

At least one brand has opted for individually wrapping each strip in foil. It's nice for keeping each one at optimum quality, never exposing it to the elements until you are going to use it, but all that unwrapping can get tedious, especially if you test a lot.

The third part of the meter trilogy is the lancing device. Often vaguely pen-shaped, this is a spring-loaded plastic mechanism whose job it is to poke a small hole in your epidermis (*fancy word for skin*), with minimum pain.

If you just rolled your eyes and said, *Yeah, right,* you are not using it correctly.

In the old days you had to be manly and just jab your finger with a needle. Yikes! Lord knows I'm not manly enough for that! The modern lancing device works like a….like a….well, kinda like a sewing machine. It very, very, very quickly advances a small needle called a *lance* outwards and then retracts it nearly instantly. The goal is to prick your finger sooooo fast your nerve cells won't even know what happened.

Most lancing devices have a variable depth gauge that controls how far the needle shoots out (or put another way, how far it shoots *into* you). The number of levels varies depending on the model, with five and nine being the most common. Low numbers are for dainty Southern debutantes whose fingers live in silk gloves. Higher numbers are for calloused Canadian lumberjacks. Most of us are somewhere in the middle.

The goal is to get blood with no pain. Or minimum pain, anyway. Now, the FDA has approved lots of meters for *alternate site testing*. That means you can test from the forearm or leg or palm rather than the finger tips. However, the AUTHOR has not approved alternate site testing. The fingertips are where the action is. They are at the cutting edge of changes in your blood sugar. Alternate sites are not as accurate in terms of up-to-the-moment information. Why test if you're not going to get the best info possible? Even the literature that comes with alternate site meters will tell you to use your fingertips when you are low.

My feeling is, don't get into bad habits.

The pad of the finger has more nerve endings than the sides or tippy-top. The tippy-top has more nerve endings than the sides. Ergo: if your fingers are sensitive, test along the side, parallel to the fingernail. Avoid the little finger, but otherwise don't play favorites. Hit a slightly different area on a different finger each time you test.

It is generally accepted that you do *not* need to use alcohol pads to clean your fingers before testing anymore and that, in fact, doing so may mess up your results.

The folks that make the lances will tell you to replace the needle every time you use it. Of course they do, they are in the business of selling you lancing needles. The truth is, you can use it many more times. How long? It depends how tough your hide is and how often you test. I know one girl who uses a needle for a year. That's extreme. I say use it until it hurts, then you know it is getting dull. For most folks anywhere between a week and a month is the lifespan for a lance. Odds are you'll accidentally stab yourself when you change the lancing needle; if you do, go ahead and check your blood sugar. No point in wasting a perfectly good drop of blood.

By the way, most, but not all, lances are compatible with most, but not all, lancing devices. Both the round ones that look like .22 caliber rifle rounds and the squarish ones with the funny little circle on the top will work with each other. The very flat ones will only fit in their own special devices.

The lances do come in various needle diameters (called *gauge* in the medical world). So if you are very young or very old, a very thin lance will be better for you. Gauge numbers are inversely proportional—the smaller the number, the larger the needle.

Once you poke a hole in your finger, a very gentle squeeze should bring the blood to the surface. If you have to milk your finger like a cow you need a deeper or larger diameter hole. Lots of pumping of the finger mixes interstitial fluid (water between cells) into the blood sample and will throw off your results.

If you have a hard time getting blood from your fingertips you can shake your hands at your sides for 30 seconds, rub your fingertips quickly back and forth on your forearm for friction-generated heat, or if your circulation is bad, hold your fingers under warm water for a half minute.

If it hurts to lance your finger, you probably have your device set too deeply or you put the clear cap on the lance. Yeah, that's for testing on your forearm. Throw the clear cap away and put the solid one on. For what it is worth, there are some folks out there who really do have hyper-sensitive fingers. For you folks there are two pretty expensive solutions: a computerized lancing device that lets you micro-control hundreds of different depths; and a laser that burns a painless hole in your skin. They do hurt the pocketbook rather than the fingertips, but you need to test and

I don't want you to suffer every day. And think how much money you'll save by not having to pay for kidney dialysis!

Using the meter in the "trenches"

So let's check our blood sugar. Right now.

OK. Are your hands clean? If you just ate a banana or had your fingers in the cake frosting it will throw your readings off. One of my Peer Educators once took a reading after eating a banana, thought he was very high—which he wasn't—took some fast-acting insulin to bring himself down. He nearly killed himself.

You don't really need to use an alcohol pad. The best thing is to wash and dry your hands. If you are out in the world, just suck on your finger for a quick moment. So long as you don't have a lollipop in your mouth this will get any residual sugar off your finger. Get out a strip and put it in your meter. If you do this before you use the lance it makes life a little easier. Strip ports tend to be at the top or at the bottom of the meter. Most modern meters don't even need to be turned on. Putting the strip in wakes them up. Make sure you know what side up the strip goes, and which end goes in.

Lance your finger, gently squeeze until you've got a nice drop of blood.

One major strip type draws blood from either side of the strip, but the vast majority draw from the tip. **Important: do not put the blood on the strip.** Let the strip drink the blood like a little vampire bat. Hold the meter/strip at a 45 degree angle to the drop of blood and gently touch the tip of the strip to the drop. *Slurrrrrrrrrp!* Most strips have a "preview" window and you can watch the blood zip up into the strip. It is **important** that this entire window be filled. If it is not, the strip doesn't have enough blood and might give a bad reading. Most meters will give you the result in 5-15 seconds.

We'll talk about how to understand the numbers in a minute, but if you get some really wild, unexpected reading, take another reading. Something really wild and unexpected might be going on; or maybe you got a "bad" strip. Always double-check unusual readings.

What do I do with the leftover blood, you ask? Most of us T-1s just lick the blood off our fingers. Most T-2s get grossed out with that technique. Some keep a Kleenex in their meter bags to dab the finger off. I've seen others use their socks! Whatever works for you. There is no right or wrong way to get rid of the extra couple million red blood cells that you didn't use.

Although all meters have a memory that stores the results, it is a good idea to keep an old-fashioned paper logbook, if for no other reason than that it requires you to think about the results.

How often should I check my blood sugar?

In a perfect world you should check your blood sugar eight times per day. That's right. I said *eight*. You should check when you go to bed. This tells you how you ended your day and is important to the next check: when you first get *out* of bed. Now you know if your blood sugar rises, falls, or stays steady while you sleep.

Many T-2s suffer from Leaky Liver Syndrome. OK, I made up LLS, it's really called *nocturnal hepatic glucose release*; but I like Leaky Liver better. So a quick biology lesson: the liver is the largest organ in your body. It's located on your right side, below the lung. Anybody know what it does? It's a multitasking organ. It filters, it makes hormones, it stores the body's energy reserves, it does windows and it makes cappuccino….

OK, sometimes I go too far. Let's focus on the energy reserve part of the liver's job. The liver is a giant sugar battery. It holds glucose to be released between meals to keep the cells fed, and in emergencies when more energy is needed. Like when you are being chased by a tiger. Hey, it could happen.

If you suffer from Leaky Liver there is really nothing physically wrong with your liver. The liver is just getting some signals crossed. It thinks the body needs sugar when it doesn't. If you routinely wake up with blood sugar higher than when you went to bed you've got LLS and there are medications for that.

If you don't test at bedtime and rising you'll never know what that tricky liver is up to when you're asleep.

In a perfect world you'd also test before and after every meal. You test after to see what effect the meal had on your blood sugar. You test before to put the after-meal score into perspective. An after-meal number by itself won't tell you very much if you don't know if it's higher, lower, or the same as the pre-meal reading.

Also, for those of us using fast-acting insulin with meals, the two-hour-after reading is our advanced warning system for low blood sugar. More on that later.

Some of the finger sticks can be combined. If you eat breakfast shortly after you get up, your rising check and your pre-breakfast check can be one-and-the-same.

Of course, very few diabetics can afford to buy the strips the insurance companies are refusing to cover. If you are in this not-enough-strips-boat, take the shotgun approach. Day one check breakfast, day two lunch, day three dinner, day four sleep and rising, rinse and repeat.

So you can understand what your doctor is telling you about blood sugar testing patterns, let me give you another quick lesson in MedSpeak.

AM Fasting: a blood sugar check before your feet hit the floor in the morning.
AC meals: before eating a meal (from the Latin *Ante Cibum*).
Postprandial: after eating, typically two hours downstream from the first bite (not the last bite), sometimes abbreviated PP.
HS: hour of sleep.
Random: any test that really doesn't fit into the other categories.

The numbers and what they mean

First, let me say a number is just a number. It is not an indictment of you as a person or an indicator of whether or not you are a "good" or "bad" diabetic. Don't let any number, or chain of numbers, get you down. Let them *empower* you.

Where should your numbers be? Like everything else in diabetes, there is not a 100% agreement on that issue amongst experts in the field. Most of the experts agree that under 115 mg/dl is where your blood sugar ought to be in the morning when you wake up: your fasting glucose. Some clinicians want it closer to 100. Depending on your meds, we really don't want you too much below 90. After you've had something to eat we look toward the period of time two hours after you chow down. If you only test before you eat you are missing out on the important part of the game: how your meds help you to deal with sugar. The whole point of testing before the meal is to have a baseline for how much you go up after eating, which is what's really important.

By the same token, if you only checked after meals it would be worthless. If you are 225 two hours after eating, should we be horrified? Well, yeah, if you started out at 118. But if you started out at 205, the meal itself went pretty well, but there is a baseline medication problem that needs to be addressed.

It is this after-meal number that is most hotly contested by various D-Experts, with opinions ranging from 140 on the low side to 200 on the high side. I tell our patients to shoot for 150 but not to worry if some meals clock in at 180. I think if you are routinely above 180 two hours after a meal, you need to look at changing what you eat, or what meds you take, or both.

How low can you go?

Low blood sugar is called *hypoglycemia*, or *hypo* for short. Generally, but not always, hypos only happen to diabetics who are on certain medications. Insulin and some pills can cause hypos if there is not enough blood sugar for them to play with. This can happen because you took too much medication, ate too little food, had more than your usual amount of exercise, or because the moon was in Virgo, the wind was from the northwest and…

Hypos are the cost of doing business with some meds, especially insulin. A properly controlled insulin-using diabetic can expect two hypos per month. If you have more than that, you are over-medicated.

A hypo is defined as any blood sugar under 75. Most people lose consciousness south of 50; but this is highly individualized and not always the same for every person every time. Hypos can hit terrifyingly fast. I one time went from 156 to 40-something in less than 5 minutes. On the bright side, they gave me a heated pillow in the Emergency Room. Nothing like a heated pillow to convince you that everything will be OK. If you go too low, you will have a seizure, pass out, and possibly die or get brain damage. It is the sugar equivalent of drowning. Brain cells begin to die pretty quickly without their food.

Every diabetic should know the warning signs of a low starting to hit. The symptoms vary but some common ones include the sensation of being in a falling elevator, dizziness, sudden sweatiness, especially around the face, shaking hands, and overall stupidity. Yep. It's true. When your blood sugar drops, so does your IQ.

I once had a bad hypo at the back of a Sam's Club. I took glucose tablets, but they didn't turn it around. I headed to the snack bar for soda and a giant cookie… but first stood in line to pay for the paper plates my wife had sent me for. I know dozens of other D-folk who've done equally bone-headed things when hypo.

It's worth mentioning that if you've been very high for a very long time, like many newly dx'd T-2s; you can suffer relative hypoglycemia. You can have the symptoms of a low even when you are really still too high. This is because your body has gotten used to being high. If this happens you **should** still treat the low even though you are in no real danger of passing out. Why suffer needlessly?

Treating any low is simply a matter of taking on some sugar. All D-folk should carry glucose tabs or some hard candy. Chocolate, although good for the soul and possibly the heart, is a poor choice to cure a hypo. Chocolate has too much fat; it will move into the blood too slowly. Juice or half a regular soda will also turn most hypos around.

The official rule is called *The Rule of 15*. Take on 15 grams of sugar, then wait the longest 15 minutes of your life and re-test. If your numbers have started to move up, do nothing more. If your numbers are flat or lower, eat another 15 grams. It is easy to over-eat a low and send yourself too high. We call this a *rebound excursion*, and it is almost as bad for you as the low itself.

If you go even lower than stupid you'll start acting drunk. Lord only knows how many diabetics have been tasered by the police and thrown into jail when hypo because they were mistaken for drunk or drugged individuals.

Which makes this the perfect place to remind you to put on and always, always, always, always wear your medical alert jewelry. There are a million to choose from out there ranging from dainty and ladylike to sufficiently macho for even the most testosterone-rich jock. Not having all that much testosterone myself, I wear sort of an art deco pendant. I sleep with it, shower with it, wear it to work and play. I never take it off so I always know it is on.

You can get necklaces, bracelets, and watches. You can mix and match to your wardrobe if you want to, but most of us are better off settling on one and treating it as permanent. As if it were a tattoo. **This one thing can save your life.** Shop around and get one you like, you're going to spend a lot of time with it. Don't be afraid to treat yourself. But hey, even if you are really poor and spent nearly your last dollar on this book (I thank you, my wife thanks you, my child thanks you, as does my publisher) you can still find simple under-ten-bucks medical alert jewelry at any drugstore.

It doesn't need to be highly detailed. All it needs to say is "diabetic." The EMTs will know what to do.

How high can you get?

High blood sugar is called *hyperglycemia*, or *hyper* for short. If you are a T-1, anything above 300 for any length of time is….dangerous. T-1s walk a mortality tightrope. Too high you die. Too low you die. In the past it was accepted that T-2s just don't go into comas on the high end; but recently we're finding that's just not the case. You have to be higher longer, but you T-2s can check out on the high end too.

The body's cells are survivors, like wolves that will chew off their paws to escape a trap. If they can't get glucose for long enough (when your *Blood Glucose Level*, or BGL, is very high there is either not enough insulin or a ton of it with car keys—either way your cells start to starve) they will start to burn fat. The by-product of this is *ketones*, a waste product damn hard to get out of the body. The pH of the body begins to change, your blood becomes more acid. The process is called *Diabetic Ketoacidosis*, or DKA for short; one of two kinds of diabetic "coma."

It takes many hours, but it can and will kill you if untreated. Signs that it is coming on are nausea and a fruity-smelling breath. Get thee to a hospital.

In many cases T-2s can walk around for months with blood sugars above 500 without going DKA. Sometimes they don't even know they have diabetes. Sometimes they know but don't want to test (you know who you are!). Even though they are walking around, they are in fact, zombies. Just because you can function does not mean your body isn't dissolving.

High blood sugar kills. It damages every internal organ. You can walk around at 500; you can be so used to it you don't even recognize you feel like shit. At the clinic, when we succeed in getting patients back down, they are amazed by how much more energy they have.

Yep, you can walk around right up until your kidneys fail or you go blind.

Ironically, perhaps perversely, the higher your blood sugar goes, the more hungry you feel. This is one of the rare times when the body's natural "feedback" system doesn't work right. You are too high. You are hungry. You eat more. You go higher.

Another common symptom of being high is that you will be… irritable. Of course, you won't notice. Your T-3 sure will. My wife tells me I get "pissy" above 200.

Two important things you need to know about your meter

"My meter is giving me an E-6 error message," said the patient.

Yeah, your test strips are expired. The meter knows this and won't work for even one hour past the expiration date. We can trick it by setting the meter to last year, and just so long as the strips aren't more than 3 months old we're OK.

"No, the strips are good for another 8 months," insists the patient, showing me the foil packet. So they are.

I take the meter and turn it on. In a few clicks I see the problem. *OK, here's the problem, your meter is set to the year 2098.*

Meter lesson number 1: make sure the date is right and the hour, if not right, is close. What happens at daylight savings time? You change your alarm clock, your VCR, the clock in your car and maybe or maybe not, the one on the microwave. Three days later you realize your watch is wrong and you fix that. But do you change the time on your meter?

It does matter. The meter has a memory because the meter companies know you don't bother to keep an actual paper logbook of your blood sugar readings. If the time is set wrong, your computerized logbook in the meter will be wrong, and all the data will be worthless.

Many doctors' offices download your meter into their computers to analyze your test results. The quality of the programs from different meters varies quite a lot, and can lead to trouble. One issue is that most, but not all, of the programs assume you eat at the same time every day. If you've told the software that breakfast is 8am then the program assumes any finger stick from 7:59 or earlier is a fasting test and any finger stick from 8:01 or later is a random or postprandial. Of course, most of us aren't that precise about when we eat so the program's summarics of before and after meal readings may be waaaaaaaaaay off.

The other weakness of the software is that if you look at averages, the software doesn't care how many tests you've taken. All of the programs provide impressive-looking graphs, but you must pay attention before making a medication change based on what you are seeing. If you only check your blood sugar in the morning twice in a two-month period most of the software programs will still give you a "two-month average" for morning blood sugar. It counts the two times you tested. It doesn't consider the 58 times you didn't.

Meter lesson number 2: calibrate. At this time there are only a few meters that self-calibrate, but this will no doubt be more common in the future. What is this *calibration* thing all about, you ask? There are manufacturing variances in test strips that can make the results quite different from batch to batch. Rather than make the manufacturing process more precise and reliable, meter companies have devised a cheap work-around. Every batch of test strips is given a code. The code tells the meter how bad the batch of strips is, and by how much to change the reading to get the results in the same general neighborhood as correct.

I'm sure it will ruin your day to learn that for the FDA to consider a test strip accurate it must be within 20% of correct. That means if your blood sugar is really 100, any test strip that reads from 80 to 120 is considered accurate and can be approved. If you don't believe me take your meter and do two tests in a row from the same drop of blood. See?

There are several ways that meters and strips talk to each other for calibration purposes. The two most common are chips and direct-entry. Meters that use chips have a removable chip the size of a dime that comes inside each box of strips. As most boxes of strips have two vials and only one chip, trouble is common. The other type requires you to enter the code using the keypad on the meter. Every time you use the meter it flashes the code at you to remind you to check to see if the vial and the meter are using the same code number.

The problem is, you see the code every frickin' time you test, but you only change it once every 100 tests. Diabetics tend to get tunnel vision. I see a lot of calibration errors.

How far off will your meter be if calibrated wrong? Depends on the meter. I've seen cases of 100 or 150 points off. If I find a patient's meter mis-calibrated I don't even look at the numbers or the log. They are too likely to be wrong.

Go. **Check your meter and your strips**. Right now. I'll wait for you.

…..
…..
…..
…..
…..
…..
…..
…..Done?

I'm guessing about half of you readers have just discovered you're having a bad day.

Where does your meter live?

Let me ask you this: if you were a soldier in a war zone, would you leave your rifle back at the barracks when you went on patrol? Yeah. I thought not. By the same token, your meter does you no good in your underwear drawer.

If you are going to use your meter to its best advantage (and why wouldn't you?) you need to have it with you. All the time. Always. No exceptions.

How you carry your meter depends on your sex and your lifestyle. Men can get a belt case for the whole kit: meter, lance, strips. Some women always carry a purse. You need to find a way that works for you, but don't go into battle without your best weapon.

That's plan "A."

Plan "B" is to have a weapon wherever you go. I have a meter on my nightstand. One in my car. One in my wife's car. One at my desk at home, one on my desk at work. If I went to the gym, which I don't, I'd have one there too.

The disadvantage of Plan "B" is that your data is all over the place. It is harder to download into a computer and study what is going on with your body and your diabetes. But it is better than going into battle unarmed.

Checkmate—the meter as the best weapon to master your diabetes

Meters matter. That is the bottom line. Some recent research out of the UK suggested that there was very little difference in control between D-folk who test and those that don't. The problem with the study is that all of the participants had undergone frontal lobotomies. *OK, that last part was black humor.*

But here is the deal, straight talk, no bullshit. Your meter has no brain. You need to use your own. If you just check your sugar and say, "well, what can I do?" it will do you no good. The meter gives you *information*. You must *use* that information.

The meter will tell you if your meds are working.

The meter will tell you what foods you can tolerate.

And which ones you can't.

You must understand that a "bad" number is not a *punishment*; it is *empowerment*. Diabetes is unique amongst chronic illnesses, well, unique amongst all diseases, in that you are in the driver's seat. It is one of the few self-managed diseases. You are the master of your fate. Your doctor is not in charge. You are. Your meter is the best and most important tool to help you understand and control your diabetes.

Some diabetics don't like checking their blood sugar. The smart ones wish they could get their paws on more strips. The more you test, the more you know. The more you know, the better your control. The better your control, the fewer your complications. The fewer your complications, the longer and sweeter your life will be.

Rejoice in checking your blood sugar.

Summary

So to review the most important things to know about your meter and using it, I've plagiarized from the Bible. Here are the Ten Commandments of Meters:

1) Thou shalt set the time and date of thy meter to the time zone and era in which thou livest.
2) Thou shalt calibrate thy meter.
3) Thou shalt test often.
4) Thou shalt test at various times of the day and night.
5) Thou shalt not be a wimp and thou shalt test on thy fingertips at all times.
6) Thou shalt think about thy numbers.
7) Thou shalt not take any number personally.
8) Thou shalt not allow thyself to go too high nor too low.
9) Thou shalt replace thy meter every three years.
10) Thou shalt carry thy meter with thee always.

Your target numbers are:

90-115 when you wake up in the morning or before a meal.
Around 150 most of the time, two hours after a meal.

Write these numbers down, memorize them, then eat the paper. And check your blood sugar two hours later.

Beyond meters

As you may or may not know, we are on the cusp of one of the biggest revolutions in diabetes since the humble meter came out back in 1980. There are devices available today that can track your blood sugar all the time in real time. They are called *Continuous Glucose Monitors*, or CGM for short.

I'm a CGM pioneer. I've worn a CGM since shortly after the first one was approved by the FDA. I think I was once told that I was the 30th diabetic in the nation to get one. Over time, I've worn four different models, so I know quite a bit about these systems. Maybe too much, but I want to try to talk briefly about them here.

Here's how they work: you insert a sensor under your skin, where it can stay anywhere from several days to a week depending on the model. This sensor is parked in your interstitial fluid—the water between your cells. So the sensors don't technically measure blood glucose at all, they measure body fluid glucose, which is really pretty darn close.

The sensor connects to a transmitter that beams data wirelessly to a pager-sized receiver. The monitors display not only the latest "blood sugar" reading, but also a line-graph of a varying number of hours. This gives you data in context and in perspective. Once you get the hang of it, it can be very empowering. Or overwhelming.

But think of it. You take a finger stick and you find you are at 110. Is this a good number? Maybe. Probably. But you have no context. The number exists in isolation. Now what if I told you that your BGL is 110 and dropping like a rock? That puts the number in a whole new context.

So if you wear a CGM, you can know at a glance not only your number, but how that number fits into the context of where you've been and where you're going. Your blood sugar now has rhythm and flow.

So how come everyone doesn't have one? Because insurance coverage for the new CGM systems is still spotty at best, and the damn things are pretty expensive. As time moves forward, however, coverage will increase and prices will drop.

CGMs do have their problems, and many early users got frustrated and threw their CGMs into lakes and rivers or smashed them against big rocks. At least metaphorically.

Here's the deal: you use a standard BG meter to *calibrate* the CGM. In other words, a couple of times per day you need to tell it "well the blood sugar looks like 158 to me," and then the CGM compares that to the readings it is getting from the sensor.

So a few pages ago we touched on how accurate meters are, right? So from the very get-go, you can be 20% off in different directions every time you go to calibrate the thing. Also, all of us early users were slow to understand just how long that calibration process took; when our CGMs seemed off, like during a quick-moving hypo, we threw more and more meter numbers at them and made the situation worse. Picture the poor "brain" of the CGM on your belt. It has one finger under the bathtub spigot and it is trying to figure out the temperature of the water. But you keep fiddling with the faucets before it can figure out how hot or cold the water is. The same thing is happening with your sensor and your blood sugar. You tell it, *hey our sugar is 156*. Then, just as the brain gets a sense of that, you say, *no wait a sec....it is 142*. Then, just as the brain gets a sense of that, you say, *no wait a sec...it is 138*. Then....

Additionally, there are two other factors that come into play. Measuring interstitial fluid is like alternate site testing; it is not up-to-the minute. And lastly, continuous monitors aren't really continuous at all. They test every 5 minutes or so. That's still a hell of a lot of tests, but there is a *sampling lag,* and a lot can happen in five minutes. The best way to grasp the problem of sampling lag is to consider this: if you are dropping really quickly (say 5 mg/dl per minute), how far will you fall in four minutes, 59 seconds? The answer is 25 points. Your last CGM reading was 103, but you are now at 78 and headed south. Not to beat a dead horse, but you must remember that Continuous Glucose Monitors aren't continuous at all.

All of these….issues…..can piss people off by causing the CGM numbers to lag a fair bit behind the finger stick numbers.

The truth you need to embrace in order to love your CGM is that *there is no real BGL*. If you use CGM you need to learn not to think about the numbers at all. The numbers don't matter. You need to learn to study the *flow* of the numbers. The value is in the trend, not in the isolated number.

The monitors also feature various alarms that, depending on the model, can alert you to high or low BGs in case your head is up your ass and you aren't paying attention, alert you to rapid changes in numbers (like when you are dropping quickly), and even predict high or low glucose a half hour before it happens. Scary shit, but waaaaaaay cool.

I stuck with mine through the wanting-to-smash-it-against-a-big-rock phase because even with all its faults I was safer with it than without it. I'm hypo unaware. I do not feel low blood sugar at all. The CGM keeps me safe. It keeps me alive. Like an arranged marriage, over time I grew to love her and understand her better.

CGM offers a great opportunity for understanding your diabetes and controlling it, and I expect the technology to get better and better. We only flew the Wright Flyer of CGMs a few years ago, and now everyone is mad 'cause we don't have jet fighters yet. Give it time.

As a final note on CGM, I want to warn you that it can also be depressing to see just how bad your blood sugar control really is. When you check your blood sugar at 10am and again at 4pm and you see a nice straight line between the checks, you feel pretty good. You tend to think the lines actually connect like some biological connect-the-dots game. The truth is, your blood sugar wanders around like a drunk sailor trying to find his way back to his ship from the brothel. Sometimes the sugar drifts upwards, sometimes downwards, frequently without discernable patterns. It's so messy, so organic, so damn… human.

> "I have a whimsical guide line on blood sugars: never drive under 70, never play poker under 80, never get married under 90."

James S. Hirsch, Type-1 Diabetic
Author & Journalist

Section 3—More about Blood, the Body, and Everything

Chapter 4—the A1C test and why it matters ....Page 65

This chapter covers the blood test that your doctor uses to judge your overall diabetes control. What is it? How does it work? Where should my numbers be? Why the hell does it matter, anyway? When you finish reading this chapter you'll have the answers to all these questions and more!

    How good a score do I need to pass the A1C test?................... Page 67

Chapter 5—Food and blood ....Page 73

Can you eat *that?* This chapter dives into the deep end of the food pool. How do various foods affect our blood sugar and why? What can you eat, what can't you eat? We'll talk about "carbs" and how and when to make lasting changes to your diet.

    Keeping it simple: the white food rule .... Page 75
    Scaling Everest one step at a time... Page 77

Chapter 6—Everything else and blood ....Page 81

This chapter looks at how just about everything in the universe can affect our blood sugar—from the chaos of everyday existence to exercise, pain, depression, and illness.

> Life is chaotic .... Page 81
> Working out .... Page 82
> Pain .... Page 83
> Depressing depression .... Page 83
> Cold and flu season .... Page 86
> Infectious infection .... Page 86

Chapter 7—Why less is more ....Page 89

Well, at some point every book about diabetes needs to talk about weight and obesity, right? This chapter looks at why it matters, how the pounds come on and how to take them off again.

> Fat matters .... Page 89
> How to lose it without losing it .... Page 91
> BMI is not an expensive car your doctor drives .... Page 95

Chapter 8—Beyond blood ....Page 97

Well, there is a lot more to diabetes than blood sugar. We need to worry about the pressure of our sweet-or-not-so-sweet blood. We also need to worry about some mysterious fats that float around in our blood called *lipids*. I'll also touch on a little gland in your neck that you may or may not even know you had—it often runs amuck in us D-folk. We'll do breakfast, or at least learn why we should. We'll also take a look at our eyes and our feet.

    Why blood pressure matters .... Page 97
    Why those crazy lipids might matter more .... Page 100
    Why you are a cave person and didn't even know it .... Page 104
    Why breakfast really is the most important meal of the day .. Page 107
    Love your feet and they'll love you back .... Page 108
    Here's looking at you .... Page 109

> "I'm talking to the cat at 5:29 in the morning while I test my blood sugar. Even as the result came back at 44 mg/dl, I had to laugh at the ridiculousness. But something about seeing that number made the symptoms of the low show themselves. Seeing that 44 made me notice the dampness on my forehead. I felt like I was about to burst into tears and into a fit of laughter at the same time."

Kerri Morrone Sparling, Type-1 Diabetic
(a.k.a. "Six" of SixUntilMe fame)
Editor & Blogger

Chapter 4—the A1C test and why it matters

So what the hell is this *Aay-one-see* everyone keeps talking about? In a nutshell, it is a blood test that is used to get an overall measure of how good or bad your blood sugar control is over a three-month period. The bottom line is that the better your blood sugar is controlled, the fewer complications you will suffer. The test, sometimes called HbA1c—or the glycated hemoglobin test to its friends—is the best tool we've got to see if your eating, activity patterns, and your medications are appropriate for your personal diabetes at a given time. It is not perfect (what is?) but it also lets us compare apples to apples. Changes in A1C over several test periods tell us if your diabetes is stable, getting better, or getting worse.

OK, how does it work and what do the scores mean? Quick biology lesson: you remember the red blood cell, right? The Martian flying saucer? Now, imagine a freshly fried doughnut hole being rolled across a tray of powdered sugar. As it rolls, the sugar sticks to the outside of the pastry. The same is true with your red blood cells; sugar molecules stick to their skins as they roll through your veins.

A red blood cell lives about three months, your bone marrow making replacement cells all the time. Using the magic of chemistry, we can analyze a blood sample and make some pretty darn good assumptions about the overall sugar environment that the cells live in. The A1C test provides a three-month window into the blood sugar environment simply because the oldest cell in any blood sample will be a geriatric 3-month-old fellow limping along with a microscopic walker.

Why do you need an A1C if you're testing your blood with your meter? Well, A1C gives us an average. We've taken your highs and squashed them down and taken your lows and raised them up. That's both good and bad as we'll see shortly. Let's say you are only testing once per day because you are a Type-2 on oral medications and you have Medicare. Medicare will only pay for one strip per day for those taking pills —for God's sake don't drop it in the toilet—and three strips per day for us insulin users; which in both cases is criminal and dangerous. We can sometimes get you more, but it takes some paperwork. *Ask you doctor if you can have more test strips.*

So let's say you use your one strip per day when you wake up in the morning and you clock perfect numbers every day. You never see anything above 115 and never below 98. You are a control machine! You are on the money, baby! You'll live forever!

Or maybe not.

Because you've got no idea whatsoever where your blood sugar is the other 23 hours, 59 minutes, and 59 seconds of the day. So you go eat your oatmeal, toast, and hash browns under the delusion that this is a healthy breakfast (more on that later) and your blood sugar rockets upwards to 275....and stays there....until bedtime....and as you sleep it slowly coasts downwards again. And you have no clue. This really does happen to people. Every day.

The A1C will warn us. You think you're in control, but the A1C can show us what happens between finger sticks.

How good a score do I need to pass the A1C test?

No one quite agrees on where your A1C score should be, but we all agree on where it *shouldn't* be. The scale does not look anything like the BGL numbers you are used to. For all practical purposes, it runs from 5.0 up to 14.0 where most in-house A1C machines max out. Labs can test higher, but at 14.0 your doctor will run screaming for the hills anyway, so it really doesn't matter. At that level your blood sugar is lethal and your body is slowly dissolving, just as if you had battery acid in your veins and arteries.

As a side note, many offices have in-house A1C machines that give results in six minutes. Very handy. I personally love being able to discuss the score with the patient during the visit. Other offices do a "send out." We generally do them in-house, but if we are also running other lab tests we'll sometimes piggyback the test onto the blood draw. Both are highly accurate and reliable.

So back to your score. Scores below 6.0 are usually considered to be in the non-diabetic range. At 9.0 we cross the threshold where kidney damage starts. So we can all agree that above 9.0 you are in deep shit and the higher above 9.0 that the number is, the worse off you are because A1C tests are curvilinear. Just like Category 3 hurricanes are much worse than Category 2 storms, or like 7.3 earthquakes are much worse than 7.0s, each increase in your A1C number packs a larger punch than you'd expect.

The numbers are sufficiently confusing that the ADA has introduced a new measure called eAG, for estimated average glucose. This is a formula that "translates" an A1C score into a "meter number." It hasn't been widely adopted yet and the jury is still out on how useful eAG is. I use it for some patients, but not for others, but I always like to have a lot of tools in my tool box.

If you are at 13.5, don't panic, but be worried. In other words, don't lie awake at night staring at the ceiling, but don't take your time getting your act together either. I've seen newly diagnosed patients with A1Cs in the 13s and 14s bring them into line within 6-9 months. Talk about feeling good when you go to bed at night, knowing you helped someone do that!

So, if 9.0 and up is bad, and below six is normal, shouldn't we all be as close to six as possible or even in the fives? Hmmmm....well, maybe not.

The practice guidelines from the ADA for quite some time have urged doctors to shoot for less than 7.0 as the number for considering a diabetic "in control." The Endos' big organization calls for "as close to 6 as possible without hypoglycemia," which many Endos feel isn't possible. Another practice guideline for docs calls for 6.5. Why all the confusion?

Diabetes History 101. OK, once upon a time there was a huge clinical trial called the Diabetes Control and Complications Trial. It was the first foray into discovering what really tight control means or doesn't mean. As it turns out, the lower your blood sugar, the fewer complications you develop. The results were not marginal by any means. In fact, the improvements in the study group over the control group were so dramatic that the study was shuttered early and all the control group diabetics were added to the intensely controlled group so that they could live longer.

That's what started the lower is better philosophy. Unfortunately, nothing is really that simple. I have a fit and fall in it when one of the patients I work with clocks a 5.8 A1C. Why? Because it can't be done *safely*. You cannot control your diabetes that well. If you've got an A1C below six, **you are having hypos**. And lots of them.

Remember? A1C is a game of averages. If you crash to 50 and rebound to 150 the average is 100. Right? Often low A1Cs are a warning sign of frequent hypos. Are frequent hypos a bad thing? Oh yeah.

First off, they make you feel like hell. Second off, they can kill you. Third off, if you have too many of them you will lose your ability to feel them—like me. I'm a reformed control freak…er…control enthusiast. I burned out my hypo warning system. I do NOT know when I'm going low. It's dangerous and scary.

Back to where to be. At my clinic we used the 6.0 to 6.9 score range as "in control" up until recently. At 7.0 and above you were considered out of control but we didn't begin to panic until you were above 8.0.

As I mentioned before, if you are below 6.0 we administer intravenous Twinkies and cut your meds back a bit.

Just when everyone was comfortable with that, everything changed again. My mother is still hopping mad that after years of eating margarine, which she hated, it was decided that butter was better for you after all. Well, that's just the way things go. As time passes we all learn more, understand more, and things change more.

The smoke hasn't cleared yet as of this writing, but a National Institutes of Health study called ACCORD, that was designed to push control into the non-diabetic range, was shut down early because the participants started dropping like flies. No one is quite sure why yet, but it has called into question the whole concept of low blood sugar as the Holy Grail.

Theories advanced include that maybe trying to drive diabetic blood sugars that low caused heart damage or that there might have been frequent hypos and rebounds that were hard on the heart. I can personally attest to the fact that a wicked low followed by a rebound can leave you feeling like the LAPD just beat the crap out of you. If you can *feel* it, it must being having *some* effect on your body. Or maybe it was just the stress of trying that hard to control blood sugars that gave people heart attacks. Who knows?

Let me tell you the tale of two patients. We've got a T-1 who is in the final, advanced stages of kidney failure. His A1C is 6.2. *WTF?* you ask. Ahhh, but you must look at his meter download. He has hypos into the 20s. Sometimes his meter says "Hi" and it's not just being friendly (in this case that means over 500). For years and years and years his "perfect" A1C scores covered up the fact he had no frickin' idea what he was doing. He was never properly instructed on how to care for his diabetes. Sloppy medical "professionals" just looked at his A1Cs and told him to keep doing what he was doing. And he did. Now it is too late.

Second patient: Type-2 with an A1C in the high 8s for years, and years, and years with no hint whatsoever of any trouble. His meter shows his BGLs are remarkably stable. Always high, but always stable. Hmmmmmmmmm….

As continuous monitoring goes mainstream *I think* we will find that within the sub 9.0 range, *excursions* will play a larger part in causing problems than average blood sugar will. "Excursion" is a word for rapid changes in blood sugar, upwards.

So you eat the fudge-fudge walnut brownie sundae at the Elephant Bar, a carb-packed creation originally designed to provide dessert for an entire African village for a week. Of course you eat the whole thing yourself. In fifteen minutes. Yes, guilty as charged, I have actually done this….but only in the interest of clinical research, of course.

And of course, your sugar explodes upwards…125…159…173…206…282…341…414…

You just had an excursion. Now if you're a T-1 like me, you took insulin before you ate that monster. A lot of insulin. But the body, medicated or not, can't deal with that kind of sugar load. Usually, 3-4 hours after an excursion you are back in normal range, but…well, we are still trying to understand the details, but it sure looks like excursions may be damaging to cellular tissue, probably causing micro-vascular damage. In other words, damaging your capillaries. Time and scientific research will tell us more. In the meantime, I can attest to the fact that if I've had a bad excursion I feel like crap; my body is sending me a message that I'd be wise to heed.

But enough of an excursion about excursions, let's get back to the A1C. Until we know more, for now I think if your A1C is between 6.5 and 7.5 you should consider yourself in control. And you should strive for stable numbers that change slowly from hour to hour.

An A1C test is run quarterly, twice a year, or once a year, depending on how good or bad your control is; how good or bad your insurance is; and your provider's approach to diabetes care.

Even in healthy, well-controlled patients, I like to run the test every quarter. If something is starting to change I want to jump on it right away. Remember: all diabetes is chronic and progressive and the body eventually adapts to all meds; they will lose their effectiveness. One of the few constants in the universe is that your diabetes will get worse no matter how hard you try. But remember, that is not a death sentence by any means. Diabetes gets worse, but we have a never-ending supply of tools to meet the menace and keep it in check.

Diabetes really isn't that hard to control; but it does, to paraphrase Thomas Jefferson, require eternal vigilance.

Chapter 5—Food and blood

"Do you have a list of foods I'm allowed to eat?" is the most common question I get from newly dx'd patients. No and we don't use leeches or bleeding anymore either. In the dark ages *and unfortunately still at many clinics,* diabetics were given draconian diets—lists of foods they were "allowed" to eat and lists of foods that were prohibited.

The problem is that it is easier to change your gender than your diet. And realistically, any medical professional that asks patients to change their diet is also either—at best—requiring the entire family to change or—at worst—creating jealousy, anger and resentment.

The fact is, a diabetic can eat anything the rest of the population can. Including cake, ice cream, candy bars and soda pop. Are those things good for diabetics? No, of course not. Are they good for non-diabetics?

I rest my case.

The only thing I ever ask patients to give up is liquid sugars such as regular soda. It is liquid poison. Serving sizes have gotten larger, and larger, and larger, and super-larger over the years. Some people fill cups that hold nearly a gallon of soda. That is more sugar than any diabetic pancreas can handle. Or any non-diabetic pancreas for that matter. And to top it off, as a complete side note, that much soda has more calories than you need for an entire meal with ZERO nutritional value.

Honorary members of the liquid sugar family include sports drinks, energy drinks, some drinks claiming to be juice, and sugar in coffee or tea. Coffee and tea are easy to fix. Instead of sugar use one of the three common artificial sweeteners: Splenda, NutraSweet, or Equal (a.k.a. the yellow stuff, the pink stuff, or the blue stuff). One of the three will appeal to your taste buds. Next time you eat out, swipe a few of each for further study at home. Just don't wipe out the entire supply; odds are the next guy to use your table has diabetes too.

Sugar-free sodas do take some time to get used to. Most folks need about two weeks to acclimate to them. Once you do, however, regular soda tastes nasty! Diet sodas do not raise your blood sugar. Oddly, however, there is quite a bit of evidence that they can cause you to gain weight. No one understands this, as there are no calories, so....*WTF?* Two possible theories are that maybe the caramel coloring in many drinks has some sort of effect; or it is possible that people who drink lots of soda have a greater propensity to having a sweet tooth and are therefore more likely to be into the Twinkies when no one is looking. The jury is out on the why, but we can see it *does* happen.

Diet, in this case meaning what we eat to survive rather than some fad eating plan to lose weight, is tricky. Entire libraries of books have been written about healthy eating and diabetes. The most important thing to remember is not to listen to your mother or your aunt or your grandma.

Like they say with cars: your mileage may vary. We are all unique. Diabetes affects each of us in different ways; but some general rules apply. First, meet the carbohydrates. Known fondly as "carbs," these are simple sugars. Foods that turn into glucose frightfully fast in your body.

Any packaged food will have its carbohydrate content listed on that little box you never read on the back. As a general rule a healthy man can tolerate a maximum of 60 carbs per meal and a healthy woman 50. Of course, technically, we D-folk aren't really healthy, now are we?

I'm extremely sensitive to carbs, so I can only tolerate 15 or so at a time without a serious excursion. If I want to keep my blood sugar in line I need to eat lots of small, healthy, lowish-carb snacks. Most diabetics fall somewhere in between—they can handle more carbs than I can, but less than a non-diabetic person. Use your meter to see how various carb counts affect you personally.

The most wicked carb in the world (and a leading cause of the obesity epidemic) is high fructose corn syrup. High fructose corn syrup is cheaper than sugar. It appears in candy, soda, and even hamburger buns. There are no high fructose corn syrup trees in nature. That, incidentally, is one of my dietary rules of thumb: the closer to the tree, the better. Which is just a way of saying that the less processed a food is, the better it is for your body. Ever heard of enriched wheat flour? Yep, it's been so heavily processed it no longer has any nutritional value at all. It is powdered library paste. They've had to put food value *back* in, thus *enriching* it.

Keeping it simple: the white food rule

So rather than give our patients a box of leeches, some bleeding blades, and a list of foods that they can't eat; I teach them the White Food Rule: *you need to moderate—not eliminate—any food that is white.*

White foods include anything made with sugar (or that nasty corn stuff), flour, rice, and potatoes. So sugar gives us candy, cake, soda, and many breakfast cereals. Flour gives us bread, tortillas, muffins, and pasta. Rice in all its various forms (brown long-grain better than white or short grain). Potatoes includes baked—which will turn to glucose in your blood faster than spoon-feeding yourself table sugar—French fries, mashed, chips, and hash browns. By the way, corn—although yellow—is an honorary white food.

These are all foods that should make up less than a third of your meal. Experiment, but in general between half a cup and one cup of any of these is the most your blood sugar will tolerate in a given meal.

Also important: take on only one white food per meal. If you want dessert, have a pork chop with green beans and a salad. If you want a baked potato with your steak, skip dessert.

You can eat anything you want. You just have to be smart about what you eat with what. Which brings me back to oatmeal, as promised.

There is nothing really wrong with oatmeal. But it is a carb. And most people sprinkle a little bit of dry, crystal carb on top. Then pour *white* carb-laden milk onto it. And eat it with white toast. Maybe they have a little fruit to be healthy. Carb attack!

That leads me to fat. Actually, fat is sometimes a good thing. (By the way, avoid "fat-free" foods. Most have heaps more sugar in them.) Two things slow down the absorption of carbs and you can use them to your advantage. One is fat, both animal and vegetable. The other is fiber.

If I eat even the smallest bowl of cereal my blood sugar will go through the roof within fifteen minutes. But, if I stir in some walnuts or eat some bacon with it, the excursion is much slower. The downside of fat of course is that if you plug up your arteries you'll drop dead from a heart attack. There you'll be on the sidewalk dead as a doornail, your blood sugar perfect.

Which brings us to the fact that there is more to diabetes than just blood sugar. Diabetes doesn't like to play alone. It brings its friends over: hypertension (high blood pressure), hyperlipidemia (high cholesterol), thyroid problems…the list goes on. But more about that in a later chapter.

Scaling Everest one step at a time

I have been accused of having an extraordinarily radical approach to diet, but I can defend myself with one simple fact: *my way works*. Let me tell you more.

In medicine we have a technique called *titration*. It is most commonly used for medications, including some diabetes meds. You start off with a little tiny bit and add more as the patient's body can tolerate it. Much like climbers going up Everest, you take it a little at a time and rest at each stage before going on.

I am a firm believer in diet titration. Here, because we are in New Mexico and 80% of our patients are Hispanic, we jokingly call it winning the war one tortilla at a time. (Political correctness note: the northern New Mexico descendants of Spanish explorers and colonists prefer the term *Hispanic* over *Latino* or any of the other classifications that are commonly used for this gene pool.)

A lot more than nutrition happens when we eat. Meals are often the focal point of family interaction. So eating is social. Meals are when we share our days and talk. So eating is news. Meals are often relaxing. So eating is soothing. Meals are often a feast for the senses—smell, taste, texture. So eating is sex.

Who the hell wants to change all of that?

Let's go back to the beginning of the book. Back to the day you were diagnosed as a diabetic. I'll wager money that many of you were given, that day or at the next visit, a list of things you could and couldn't eat. You probably tried your level best. You wanted to be healthy, for yourself, for your family. Maybe you like your doctor and didn't want to let him or her down.

But….

But maybe your family wasn't on board with you on that food list.

But maybe you found that your meals became lonely, newsless, tense, and sexless. You probably tried for months. One day you said, *screw it*. And in the back of your mind your inner voice was still calling *Diabetes? I can't have diabetes! I feel fine!*

You probably went back to your doctor a few more times; but the staff was rude to you about your blood sugar numbers. (They might have even called you a *non-compliant* diabetic. They did not understand. This is why everyone who works for me is either diabetic or T-3; I believe that you really need to walk in our shoes to help or even be credible.) So at some point you stopped going to your doctor.

They did you a mis-service bordering on unintentional malpractice. They asked you to go a bridge too far. They asked you to walk up Everest without stopping to acclimate.

I once had a run-in with one of our Nurse Practitioners. We had a mutual patient who, kid you not, drank 12 beers per day. She told him he had to quit, right there, right then. Cold turkey.

That may have been medically sound advice, but not humanly possible. This guy is not a machine. He is a person who lives in a complex social environment. He has deeply ingrained habits. It was too far to go. I told the NP we'd be lucky ever to see the guy again.

We were lucky. He didn't come to see her again, but he came to see me. "She told me I had to quit my beer," he told me, "I just can't. I'd rather die."

OK, I told him, *I don't really give a shit about the beer. Yeah, it's not that good for your liver or your weight; and it'll make controlling your blood sugar a little harder....but we can work around it. Hey, could you kick just one beer a day to the curb for me?*

And one beer…he could walk that far. In another month two beers were gone. Then three. He's still drinking more in a day than I drink in six months, but he's improving. We'll get there.

The Practitioner wanted all or nothing. I think too often we end up getting nothing. I'm all for slow and steady wins the race. I guess it's the classic tortoise and hare thing.

So as to what you eat: make slow steady changes. Acclimate. You'll get to your goal in the fullness of time. Better late than never—and I would argue that with diet change those are the only two options.

Each little change you make that improves your blood sugar or weight will make you feel better. That will give you the motivation to take the next step.

Chapter 6—Everything else and blood

What else affects my blood sugar, you ask? Why, everything of course! What do you know about Chaos Theory? Yeah, I don't know much either, I can't even balance my checkbook. But as I understand it with my third-grade grasp of mathematics, Chaos Theory is a way of explaining the interactions of events in complex environments with lots of variables. It's the whole a-butterfly-flaps-its-wings-in-Mongolia-so-it-rains-in-Flagstaff kind of science.

Life is chaotic

As a diabetic, I guarantee that you live in a complex environment full of variables. Sure, what you eat has the greatest effect on your blood sugar; followed closely by your patterns of activity (read exercise in the broadest sense of the word). But you are not a machine. You are a complex organism made up of over 50 trillion individual cells dancing together in a divine cosmic dance. As the music changes so does the dance. Sometimes slow and romantic, sometimes elegant, sometimes break-dancing. Your body is also coursing with hormones and filled with electricity. Sound like chaos?

What affects your blood sugar? Stress. Lucky none of us suffer from that, huh? Caffeine. If you are female, your period affects your blood sugar. If you are male, your lady's period affects your blood sugar. The weather affects your blood sugar. If you've hurt yourself, pain affects your blood sugar.

Sometimes patients will despair over a mystery spike on their meter. They did everything right and still clocked a 325. I'll kid that *the Moon is in Mercury, the barometric pressure is dropping, the wind is from the west, so of course your blood sugar did the funky chicken dance.* But at the same time, I'm not really kidding at all. All the million little things that affect our bodies, the Chaos we live in, affects our blood sugar. There are too many variables to even comprehend, much less control.

We do the best we can; but when it all goes wrong, just eat cheesecake. Forget it and move on. That said, there are a few things you can generally count on.

Working out

Exercise generally lowers blood sugar, sometimes for hours, unless you're doing some sort of crazy adrenaline-driven power exercise. The perfect exercise is one which is integrated into your day rather than a planned workout. Throw away your forged Handicapped placard and park way the hell out by the street when you go to Wal-Mart. Use the stairs, not the elevators. Take a short walk at lunch every day.

How much you should exercise depends on your goals and your health. Everyone should exercise some. Even 20 minutes per day will lower your blood sugar for 24 hours. Two ten minute walks is as effective as one 20 minute walk. Exercise is good for the body, good for the soul, good for the blood sugar, but not actually that good for losing weight. More on that in the next chapter.

So for me, talking about exercise logically leads into talking about pain....

Pain

A while back I broke my toe by violating one of the rules I always preach to my patients: never go barefoot (I think I mentioned that I'm a poor role model). Anyway broken toes, like broken ribs, hurt like hell and there is not much you can do but suffer until they heal. Guess what? Pain affects your blood sugar. So *acute* (slamming your hand in the car door), *transient* (your healing toe) or *chronic* (arthritis or fibromyalgia) pain will all affect your blood sugar, generally by raising it. When you suffer pain, your body is under assault; your caveman DNA goes into its primitive fight-or-flight mode. The result is that pain causes a constant dribble of adrenaline into your blood as long as it lasts, raising your blood sugar level. The evolutionary blueprint is that you need extra energy to recover, to fight the pain. Of course we are not in our evolutionary environment. Instead, when in pain, we lie on our couches and watch DVDs. Until we fall asleep. At least that is how I cured my broken toe.

Depressing depression

Speaking of lying on the couch watching DVDs, depression also affects your blood sugar and diabetes and depression are like inseparable high-school sweethearts. There are two reasons why virtually all diabetics battle depression to some degree or another. First, diabetes, for reasons not totally understood, physiologically *causes* depression. Not to treat anyone like an idiot, but I want to be really, really, really clear on what *physiologically* means—because many folks think depression is all in their heads. Wrong. Something that is only in your head is *psychological*. Like a fear of spiders, shopping addictions, and arranging your underwear in alphabetical order by color.

Any physiological process is more mechanical in nature; it is essential biology. A physiological process is the body working—correctly or incorrectly—independently of the brain. It is the sole province of the body itself on the most primitive level.

In our case, diabetes short-circuits something, possibly *serotonin* levels, which causes depression. Physiologically. Beyond your control. Serotonin (also called 5-hydroxytrptamine—bet you didn't know that....or care) is a hormone found in the pineal gland, in blood platelets, and in the digestive tract. See where this is going? Its actual job is as a chemical messenger between nerve cells and blood vessels to signal vessel contraction. OK, so serotonin's day job is not relevant here. But we do know that altered serotonin levels in the brain can affect mood and cause....wait for it... depression!

Look at the cast of characters here. The pineal gland is part of the endocrine system. Diabetes is a disease of the endocrine system (the pancreas is a major player in all things endocrine). Hmmmm.... And blood. And digestive tract. Is it any wonder that diabetes affects serotonin? So we know that screwed-up serotonin causes depression. And we can see that diabetes affects many of the places serotonin lives. Is it any wonder we are all depressed?

The wicked thing about depression is that being diabetic can really be depressing in the first place. It is a wearing 24-7-365 grind. Never ending. Test, test, test. Take meds. Moderate this, don't drink that. How many carbs in that Quesada? Oh crap, we've been invited to a party; I just know they are going to have a ton of sweets! My foot hurts, am I developing neuropathy? I wonder if my kidneys will fail or if I'll have a heart attack first? Damn, I forgot my meter. Did I take my pills today? *Arrrrrrrrrrrrrrrrrrrrrrrg!*

So for years I *knew* I was depressed. But I had a lot to be depressed about. Being diabetic and all. It took me a long time to realize that this was a physiological part of diabetes that needed to be fixed with medication just the way my insulin deficiency needed to be fixed with shots.

The bottom line for D-folk is that there are heavy-duty causes of depression affecting both mind and body. Most of us are on anti-depressants and the rest of us should be. There is no stigma here. We suffer from a depressing chronic, progressive illness which by itself can cause depression biologically. That's two strikes against us. We can't wait for strike three.

As to depression and blood sugar, depression causes some folk's blood sugar to go up, others' to go down. Also, if you get in a funk you will probably stop checking your BGL for days, weeks, even months. At which time you'll start to notice you don't have as much energy as you used to. Yeah, you pee a lot, but you're drinking a lot of water lately. Yeah, your vision isn't what it used to be, you'll probably need new glasses. You'll take care of that soon. Sound familiar? All symptoms of high blood sugar.

And you know, if your blood sugar is high, you'll be much more likely to catch a cold or flu bug. (Actually flu is a virus, not a bug…)

Cold and flu season

And if you are sick, will it affect your blood sugar? Of course it will. Everything affects your blood sugar. Again, your mileage may vary, but most D-folk see their BGLs elevate when they are sick. Which makes you feel even worse. And when your sugar is high it takes longer to get well and….

Infectious infection

Personally, I think that if it were a truly just universe, those of us suffering from diabetes would be immune to all else—including mosquito bites and common colds. But the truth is that diabetes and infections of all kinds exist in an odd symbiotic chicken-and-egg kind of relationship.

For instance, if you are sloppy about brushing your teeth you can get a gum infection called *periodontal disease* (first warning sign: small amounts of blood when you brush). This low-grade infection will make it nearly impossible to control your blood sugar. And if your blood sugar is all over the place it makes it nearly impossible to beat down the infection. It is a dance that can go on waaaaaaaaaaaay too long.

High blood sugar can also make healing very, very, very slow. Paper cuts can take weeks to heal in some D-folk. Be alert for infection any time you are injured and know that your blood sugar may get wacky. On the flip side of that coin, if your blood sugar gets wacky for no reason, assess your health. What? You feel totally fine? Oh, except it hurts a little when you pee? Maybe you have a urinary tract infection.

I should also mention that yeast just loves growing in high sugar environments, so diabetic females with high blood sugars are plagued with more yeast infections than their non-diabetic counterparts. Yeast infections can be stressful and painful, and we all know what stress and pain do to our blood sugars, right?

"If you take care of yourself, you will be healthier and happier than you ever were. That paradox is something many of us experience."

David Mendosa, Type-2 Diabetic
Journalist of *mendosa.com* fame

Chapter 7—Why less is more

Well, you knew I'd have to talk about the whole weight thing at some point, didn't you?

This is a delicate subject, but it does matter. We are a highly schizophrenic culture. On average, we are fat, but we worship thin. Magazines and media and Hollywood all glorify an ideal that is not only unattainable, but actually unhealthy.

Fat matters

Fat matters. Fat people die earlier. If you are fat your heart works harder. No, that's not really quite true: your heart *overworks*. Your knees give out earlier. Clinical research shows that being fat can lead to liver disease, gallstones, gout, skin trouble, chronic heartburn, arthritis, some cancers, and chronic lower back pain. That's on top of the obvious higher blood pressure, elevated cholesterol, stroke risk, shortness of breath and all of that. Plus bigger clothes cost more.

But the real fly in the ointment for us D-folk is that the heavier you are, the higher your insulin resistance. And if your insulin resistance is high it will take more meds and more hard work to keep your blood sugar in control.

So to me, as a diabetes educator, reducing insulin resistance is the supreme goal of weight loss. The facts that you'll live longer, move better, have more energy, enjoy shopping again and have better sex are all just icing on the cake.

Now I have a confession to make. I'm an *ex*-fat man. I used to be six foot two inches tall and weighed close to 250 pounds. I've now shrunk to 6 foot even and 180 pounds. Of course, the one had nothing to do with the other—I lost the inches due to osteopenia (diabetes doesn't play alone, remember?).

But the weight loss came from my diabetes and changes in my eating habits post-dx. People who didn't know the old me often call me skinny which comes as a great surprise because I was overweight both as a child and for most of my pre-D adult life. I still see a fat man in the mirror. Those who knew me as the fat man worry I'm wasting away.

As an ex-fat person I can personally attest to how much better I feel as a thinner person. The biggest thing I notice is that I have more energy. And I also don't get out of breath walking from the couch to the fridge. And my blood pressure is better. And it's easier to buy clothes.

All of that said, I try real hard not to be a weight Nazi, like those reformed ex-smokers we all know who go on a crusade to convert everyone else to their new way of life. For me, being a T-1, the weight loss wasn't really that hard.

When my Endo promoted me to T-1, I went on a mission to learn everything there was to know about my new condition. Time and time again I read how T-1s were usually described as skinny. One visit I said to her, *How come I'm the only fat Type-1 in the world?*

"Just wait," was her reply.

Sure enough, over the next few months I melted like ice cream left on the porch on a sunny summer day. No one agrees if it was the particular flavor of diabetes I have or the changes in eating that were required to survive and thrive that resulted in the weight loss. Probably some of each, I think.

But I know that for most people weight loss is very, very difficult. Even more so for T-2s. Don't forget the vicious cycle: weight gain causes an increase in insulin resistance, which causes increased fat storage, which causes more weight gain, which causes more insulin resistance, which….

So on one hand I understand how hard it is for most people to lose weight and what a struggle it can be. On the other hand, as a medical professional, I know that weight causes a whole host of problems. As always, I try to strike a humanistic balance. And like diet change, I believe one tiny step at a time makes the journey easier.

How to lose it without losing it

The line between losing weight, gaining weight, or holding a steady weight is much more razor-thin than most people would ever guess.

Dr. Francine R. Kaufman, in her book *Diabesity,* said it so well that I'm just going to quote her here:

> *"Our margin of error is very small...if you consume 10 extra calories or burn 10 fewer calories...over the 365 days of the year, you'd gain about a pound of fat. And if you make changes that amount to an excess of 100 calories per day—a latte with whole milk instead of skim would do it—you could be up 10 pounds in a year."*

Let's start with that ten calories, shall we? Can you name five foods that have ten calories?

Half of a single Nacho Cheese Dorito
Two baby carrots
Three-quarters of a Zesta cracker
Two Ghirardelli chocolate chips
Six raisins

So it doesn't really take a whole lot of excess calories (read overeating beyond your body's needs) to start packing on the pounds, huh?

Luckily the reverse is true too. Cut back 10 calories beyond your needs and you'll lose a pound in a year; 100 calories per day buys you 10 pounds. There are actually only three ways to lose weight. Well, four if you count liposuction. You can eat less, exercise more, or eat a little less and exercise a little more at the same time. Within limits, that last choice is, I think, the best. There is a reason I qualified that. The first risk is that if you go nuts and hire a personal trainer and work out 9.735 hours per day you'll probably start eating a whole lot more. The second reason is that it takes a lot more exercise than you might expect to actually lose any weight.

To lose a pound you need to burn off 3,500 calories, nearly two full days of healthy calorie intake. For perspective, if you rode your bike for 100 miles in under six hours you could burn five to six thousand calories. Assuming you didn't die of a heart attack at mile 25, and assuming you did not eat anything extra that day, you'd work off a pound-and-a-half.

What about less radical exercise?

> One hour of aerobics burns 422 calories.
> —You need 8 sessions to lose one pound.
> One hour of stationary bike burns 352 calories.
> —You need 10 sessions to lose one pound.
> One hour of walking burns 250 calories.
> —You need to walk 14 hours to lose one pound.
> One hour of weight lifting burns 211 calories.
> —You need 16 ½ sessions to lose one pound.

What about having sex? Sex burns only 80 calories. Sorry. You need to "do it" 44 times to lose one pound.

The point of all of this is that although exercise is very good for both body and soul health, it doesn't shave many pounds. Cutting calories put into your mouth is the best way to lose weight.

Let's say you want to lose 20 pounds in one year. What are your options? We need to cut or burn 70,000 calories. So for exercise you could do 166 hours of aerobics, 199 hours of stationary bike, 280 hours of walking, or 332 hours of weight lifting. Or you could have sex 875 times.

On the other hand, to lose the same 20 pounds by reducing your food intake you need to shave about 200 calories a day off your diet. If you eat three meals per day that's only 66 calories per meal. Dropping a half a slice of bread per meal would do it for many people. Bottom line, exercise does the body good in many, many, many ways, but the best way to lose weight is to simply eat less, *or better*.

How much weight should you lose? Are you a 360-pound 5 foot 5 inch 62-year-old man, or a 190-pound 6 foot 34-year-old woman? See? No simple answer. However, if you lose 7% of your body weight you will make a significant impact on your insulin resistance. But each and every pound will help. Set a realistic goal and take it one baby step at a time. Maybe you can only lose a pound a month. I'm OK with that. It's progress towards the goal, and every bit you lose, no matter how small, will make you feel that much better in every way.

A patient who is very heavy recently asked me if I thought he should consider gastric bypass surgery. I told him I thought a *refrigerator-ectomy* would probably do him more good. In all fairness, I don't know much about these stomach-shrinking surgeries. But my gut instinct is this: only go "under the knife" to save your life. You have other options for losing weight.

So my thoughts and strategies on losing weight are as follows: Never eat seconds. That said, now please do not fill that first plate with twice as much food. If you don't already eat seconds, buy smaller plates. If you go to an antique store and look at the size of dinner plates and breakfast bowls that were used 50 years ago compared to today's you'll be amazed. Eat slowly. Do NOT eat in front of the TV. Light a candle, sit at a table and converse with your loved ones while you eat. The more you talk, the less you eat. The slower you eat the more likely the signals that tell your brain that your stomach is full will get there before you overeat. Drink lots of water. Consider eating your side salad at home *before* the meal like you do at a restaurant. Remember to moderate your white foods and avoid white food stacking (you don't really need *both* dinner rolls *and* a baked potato in one meal). Anything "bad" for you that you just can't stand to do without, cut back on 10% at a time over many weeks. But never, never, never *completely* eliminate anything that you love to eat, no matter how "bad" it is for you. *Life is too short to spend it in misery.*

BMI is not an expensive car your doctor drives

As a final note on weight, I want to touch on Body Mass Index. BMI is a ratio of height to weight that, like FAX machines, is a system that was never perfected. It is supposed to give you an idea if you are underweight, just right, overweight, or dangerously obese.

But there are problems. First off, some people are built stocky. Others have more delicate frames. BMI does not compensate for body type.

Also, muscle weighs considerably more than fat does. Many bodybuilders have BMIs that would suggest they are obese when they don't have any body fat to be seen anywhere….and 'cause they're wearing Speedos there aren't too many places we can't see.

What we really need is a way to measure how much body fat a person has. The problem is, most of the methods available have more in common with witchcraft than science. So we are stuck with BMI for now. At least it gives us apples to apples comparisons on one person's progress (or lack thereof) and gives us a loose framework for comparing patients to each other. But it's a crude instrument at best; don't lose too much sleep over your BMI.

Chapter 8—Beyond blood

o as long as your blood sugar is great and your weight is OK you have no worries, right? Uh… no. Sorry. Remember that diabetes doesn't play alone?

Trivia question: what kills most diabetics? If you answered "diabetes" you must now go to the back of the classroom. Unless you were already sitting in the back of the classroom, in which case you must now come sit in the front. The answer is *heart attacks*. So it pays to keep your heart healthy.

Why blood pressure matters

When it comes to the heart, there are two things you need to watch: pressure and lipids. More on lipids in a minute. Checking your blood pressure is easy, fast, and free; so there is no excuse for only having it checked at your annual physical. Most county health offices and community clinics will do a BP check for free on a walk-in basis. So do many drugstores. Lots of mass merchants and grocery stores have free automated systems in their pharmacy departments.

You can also get an automatic home model for anywhere between $15 and $50. There is some controversy about the accuracy of home models, and some of that may come down to how well the user follows the directions for using them. I think that so long as you avoid the wrist and fingertip models and get one you wrap around your bicep (upper arm) they are worth owning.

Even if not 100% accurate, you can test at various times of the day and if you are becoming *hypertensive* (fancy word for having high blood pressure) you'll have advance warning. Hmmmm....sounds sort of like watching your blood sugar, doesn't it?

Blood pressures are expressed in two numbers. The ideal target is 120/80. OK, so what does that mean? We talked about the circulatory system earlier. You've got arteries, veins and capillaries making up an incredibly complex plumbing system for your blood. At the center of your body lies the heart, which is a pump. It fires up when you are in your mother's womb and keeps on ticking to the day you kick the bucket. It pumps by contracting to shove blood from its chambers into the arteries, then takes a quick breather, relaxes and refills, then squeezes again.

Unless you just had your arm bitten off by an alligator—hey, it could happen—your network of veins and arteries is a totally closed system. There are no openings to the outside world. Thus the system has a static pressure when the heart is at rest and a peak pressure when the heart pumps. Eureka! The two numbers in your blood pressure! The top number is the pressure when the heart is pushing a wave of blood through the system, and the bottom number is the overall pressure in the system when the heart is at rest. Obviously, the top number is always higher unless you are dead.

Side note: blood doesn't really flow through your body. It *pulses*. Picture it like a perfectly choreographed traffic jam on the freeway. All the blood cells are lined up bumper-to-bumper. When the heart beats all the cars move forward a few feet and stop. Then the heart beats again and they all jump forward a few more feet and stop. You can feel the pulses of life coursing through your own body. Take your index finger and middle finger and lay them across your wrist. Press down lightly. Feel it?

So back to pressure. My little son likes to play with balloons. Statistics on how many children choke and die each year on balloon pieces sometimes leave me lying awake at night staring at the ceiling, but he likes to see how much he can blow them up. How big can I get it without a major structural failure? In the case of a balloon, a major structural failure would be what? Yeah, it would ***pop***. Now, have you ever really put some brain power into a popping balloon? If we could see it in slow motion, what would we see?

Well, balloons aren't perfect. Somewhere on the surface there's a spot that is just a little bit thinner than the rest. Too much pressure on this spot will cause a little tiny breach. A hole. It could be the size of a pin. The air pressure inside the balloon is now much higher than the pressure in the outside world.

Nature always seeks a balance. The air inside is contained. Forced into the balloon, held tight by the balloon's walls. Like death row inmates, those air molecules want out!

The air inside the balloon rushes into the breach. In milliseconds of incredible violence the breach becomes a huge tear. The very fabric of the balloon is torn asunder by the fearsome force of nature. When this happens to a blood vessel inside the human body we call it a *stroke*.

If your bottom number is above 100, the pressure in your system is so high you are in stroke territory.

Hypertension is a tough nut to crack. There are things you can do, like lose weight, reduce the salt in your diet, and eat healthy; but in most cases you need pills. And often not just one. More and more we are finding that hypertension requires two or three meds to rein it in. To make your life easier, many pharmaceutical companies are now making poly-pills; pills that contain more than one kind of drug. *Ask your doctor if poly-pills are right for you.*

Why those crazy lipids might matter more

Now, I mentioned lipids at the start of the chapter. Lipids are, in essence, fats. There are many, but three in particular cross our radar: LDL and HDL Cholesterol and Triglycerides. Triglycerides are blood fats. Your doc will check your level with a blood draw once per year. Your target is less than 150. If they are too high the risks include coronary artery disease. That can net you a complication called *atherosclerosis*, a.k.a. hardening of the arteries (more about that in a second), which in turn leads you to a stroke or heart attack.

High triglycerides can also cause pancreatitis, an extraordinarily painful inflammation of the pancreas. High triglycerides can be treated by cutting back on certain dietary fats and alcohol, or by adding meds. By the way, if your blood sugar is high it is impossible to get an accurate reading of your triglycerides.

Thanks mainly to big Pharma's TV ads, Cholesterol is better known; but the two types are often confused. LDL is the "bad" cholesterol and HDL is the "good" cholesterol. The best way to remember the difference comes from Paula Devitt, RN CDE, of Christus St. Vincent Regional Medical Center's Diabetes Center of Excellence in Santa Fe, New Mexico, who calls LDL that "Lousy Darn Lipid." I've been known to substitute slightly harsher language for "darn."

Those Lousy Darn Lipids coat the inside of your blood vessels with plaque. Have you ever had the misfortune of replacing any old plumbing in your house? Ever look at the build-up of gunk in really old pipes? Yuck! Well, actually, the same thing happens in your body. The LDL builds up plaque on the walls of the vessels.

It can actually fill up a vessel to the point that it is occluded, or totally blocked. The blood cells get stuck, can't get through, and they clot.

And clots cause most heart attacks.

So it's pretty clear why LDL is lousy. What's up with "good" cholesterol? Remember the Dow Scrubbing Bubbles? Yep, that's HDL. They are the body's scrubbing bubbles. HDL scrubs out the plaque and keeps your blood vessels sparkly clean and free of occlusions.

Within limits, the ideal is to have your LDL low and your HDL high. For men with diabetes it is universally agreed that your HDL should be above 40 and for women above 50.

LDL targets are more controversial thanks to a lot of scary, keep-you-awake-at-night, new research that is beginning to reveal that even tiny differences in LDL scores can literally add or subtract *years* from your life.

Most current practice guidelines establish an LDL target of less than 160; but this is hotly contested with some practitioners suggesting 130, 100, or even 70! Several Lipidologists have even suggested 50 as a target for high risk patients. Who's high risk? Well, diabetics…

All of that said, most diabetic care guidelines establish goals of less than 100, or less than 70 if there is any heart attack risk. The problem with that, of course, is that all D-folk are at risk of a heart attack. Remember what kills most of us?

For what it is worth I recently attended a lecture by noted Lipidologist Dr. Michael Davidson who pointed out that most mammals have LDLs around 50. I think rats had the lowest and lions had the highest, but they were all pretty close. By the way, newborn humans have an LDL around 50 too……*hmmmmmmmmmm*….

And if all of that weren't complicated enough, there is a whole new way of looking at the cholesterol picture. There are actually quite a few more types of cholesterol that we are learning more about every day. The problem is that insurance companies don't want to pay for the tests that can ferret out their levels. Thus the medical community has come up with an elegant workaround: the Non-HDL Cholesterol.

You get this number by subtracting your HDL from your total cholesterol and adding 30 points. Where that new number should be depends on your heart risk. For the highest risk patients goal is 130 and optimal is considered 100.

For the next tier down, moderately high risk….say diabetes and high blood pressure….the goal is less than 160 and optimal is considered less than 130. Remember that those numbers are for Non-HDL Cholesterol. This won't be on your lab reports. You need to get out a calculator or slide rule!

Given the strong link between LDL and heart attacks, and the fact that heart attacks finish off most of us D-folk, I kinda think that without going overboard, we are better off looking to keep ourselves on the low side of the current guidelines.

LDL is lowered using a family of meds called statins. As an ounce of prevention, **it is now recommended that all D-folk take a statin whether or not our cholesterol is high.** For similar reasons, unless your other meds make it a bad idea, you should also take a baby aspirin every day (81 mg).

Why you are a cave person and didn't even know it

So now I want to tell you about cavemen. Oh, and cavewomen too of course. We all carry a little piece of each around in our throats in the form of the black sheep of the endocrine system: the stupid, primitive little gland called the *thyroid*.

The thyroid's job is to regulate your metabolism. As it's part of the endocrine system, it's no wonder that it often gets messed up in diabetics. Most commonly it under-performs, which paradoxically causes a high score on a blood test called TSH.

Have your doc check your TSH annually. The common wisdom is that this score should be below 4.0, and you should be medicated if higher than that. I'm here to tell you that *that* is wrong, and diabetic docs on the cutting edge maintain that it needs to be under 2.0.

The reason I want you to have it checked every year is that the leading symptom of your thyroid being out of whack is fatigue. The problem is, who isn't, nowadays? There are always reasons to justify being tired, so it often doesn't occur to us to look for a medical problem.

The name-brand thyroid med is called Synthroid. The generics are called levothyroxine. Some docs think generics are just fine, others will have a fit over the thought of using anything but the name brand. Why the divide?

Real world lesson #138: Patent Law and Pharmaceuticals. Now we tread where economics and politics meet in ethical gray waters. For the Defense the argument goes like this: we drug companies spend millions (billions, gazillions, depending on who you ask) developing our drugs. We have to test them on rats, rabbits, convicts, then volunteers. We have to buy hookers for the FDA folks. It costs us a lot of money to get a drug to market. Then we only have a limited amount of time to make back our investment and make a profit for our shareholders before our patent runs out and some guy in China can take our hard-earned recipe (without spending a dime!) and can make our drug and sell it as a cheap generic. And hey, don't forget we'll sometimes give a few bottles to some poor folks to make us look good and don't forget too that only one drug in 100 actually makes it to market. We have to support all those research projects that failed, you know. But hey, it's really all about the patient. We're not in this to make money. We only want to make people's lives better. Honest.

For the Prosecution the argument goes like this: you jackasses spend most of your money on golden parachutes for your executives and on making ads that say "ask your doctor about _____." Most drug research happens in universities and is Federally funded. If something looks promising, you buy the patent rights and run with it. You are greedy bastards who charge as much as you can in different markets, which is why a drug that costs three dollars in Canada costs thirty dollars in the States.

Like all things, there is truth on both sides. But here is the hidden fact: to be approved as a generic by the FDA, a drug must have an 80% efficacy.

That means it must be eighty percent as effective as the name brand. As far as the FDA is concerned, plus or minus 20% is OK (just like test strips!).

Oh well, if your allergy med is 80% as good as the name brand that's OK. If your cholesterol med is only 80% as good as the name brand that's probably OK. If your cough syrup, antibiotic, hypertension, and indigestion drugs are only 80% as good as the name brand, that's OK.

Not true of thyroid hormone. A tiny bit makes a big difference. Actually, you'll be OK with generic *if you always get the same brand*. The trouble is in how drugs are sold. Most pharmacies buy their drugs from big middleman distributors. On Tuesday brand A might be two cents cheaper than the others. On Wednesday it might be brand B. Drugstores even have pre-printed colorful little stickers they put on your bottles that say "Don't panic, even though your meds are a different shape and color than they were last time it's still the same medication. Really, trust us. Would we lie to you?"

If your thyroid is out of whack, only use generic if your supplier can promise you will always get the same brand. It may be off from the name brand, but it will be consistently off, and once you get it adjusted, you'll be OK.

It is important to point out that thyroid pills are the three-year-olds of pharmaceuticals. They don't play well with others. You absolutely must take your thyroid pills on an empty stomach with at least 8 ounces of water with no other pills whatsoever!

Why breakfast really is the most important meal of the day

Oh, one more thing about the thyroid. Remember the cavemen/women and metabolism? So the properly working thyroid sets the body's metabolic rate for the day. But it is a stupid, primitive, evolutionary caveman/woman throwback. If you don't eat first thing in the morning the thyroid says, "Oh crap, the clan didn't down a mammoth today. Lord only knows how long it will be until we get to eat again." And it goes into fat-storing mode.

Uh-oh.

If on the other hand, you eat breakfast, your stupid thyroid assumes that the clan brought down that mammoth and that there is plenty of food to be had. It puts you into fat burning, energy using mode.

It is a documented fact that folks who actually eat breakfast lose more weight and/or are less heavy than those who skip breakfast. I know this is counter-intuitive. We have patients who haven't eaten breakfast (or even lunch too in some cases) for years who can't see how adding *more* calories will help them lose weight.

But it is true.

Partly it is the whole metabolic thing, and partly it works like this: if you go hungry for most of the day, you eat more when you do eat. Also, pretty much anything you eat in the morning you'll burn off during the day. In a perfect world we'd eat a big breakfast, moderate lunch, and light dinner. Most Americans do the opposite. We eat our big meal in the evening, then sit on our couches and watch TV, burning very few of those calories packed on at dinner.

Love your feet and they'll love you back

Speaking of the end of the day, I tell patients to kiss their feet good night every night. That's just my way of saying get in the habit of paying attention to your feet before you need to.

Remember neuropathy? Right. That whole *you-can-lose-feeling-in-your-feet-step-on-a-nail-not-know-it-develop-an-infection-then-an-abcess-then-gangrene-then-we-cut-your-foot-off* thing. Basic rule for D-folks that we all ignore: **never go barefoot**. My real-life solution? **Just check your damn feet every night**. Run your hands over your feet every night when you get into bed. *Look* at them. If you are too hefty to see your feet get yourself a mirror.

If you get into this habit before you lose any feeling (no guarantee you will, but in this case an ounce of prevention can save you a couple of pounds of leg) *if* you have any trouble later you will be in the habit of checking; you'll find trouble if it happens.

Love your feet and they'll love you back.

Here's looking at you

OK, here is the deal. Remember all the blind D-folk we talked about in the chapter on complications? There are a couple of ways to avoid joining their ranks. The first and best is to keep your blood sugar down. That said, like most diabetic complications you don't really feel the problem until the horse has left the barn and the barn has burned to the ground.

Every year, without fail, no matter how good your A1C, no matter how good your blood sugar control is **you need to get a dilated eye exam**. And be sure to tell the eye doctor that you have diabetes.

Yeah, I hate dilated eye exams too. But ya gotta do it. So you'll stumble around like a drunk sailor while wearing dark sun glasses inside Pizza Hut. You'll be fine by the next day.

Those painful drops force the iris of your eye to open wide, like a peeping Tom watching the neighbors in the full moonlight. That lets the eye doc see the back of your retina (eye ball). He can actually *see* the blood vessels in your eyes. Cool and scary. Scarycool.

He'll look for ruptures and assorted trouble. God forbid the eye doc finds trouble, there are things you can do *before* you go blind.

Every year. Get your dilated eye exam.

"Round and round and round it goes, and where it stops could be my toes. ¶ I'd like to keep mine. Yes, that's wise. I'll keep my nerves and feet and eyes. ¶ I'd like to keep them all, mind you… So I'll do what I have to do. ¶ But like it? No, no, no, I say! I do not like the vials, the rules, the thinking, worrying all day… ¶ I do not like it one little bit. Still, I'm glad to *LIVE* with it."

Amy Tenderich, Type-1 Diabetic
(with her take on Dr. Suess)
Journalist, Advocate, Ultimate Blogger

Section 4—The Meds

Chapter 9—Doctors, medications, and you ....Page 115

In this chapter we open up the medicine cabinet and start to look at all of our options to help control our blood sugars. It also covers why it is important to understand your medicines yourself and not to rely too heavily on your doctor.

> Two flavors, not thirty-one ....Page 115
> Your partner not your boss ....Page 116
> The word "die" is part of diet..Page 118
> A kinder, gentler approach .... Page 120

Chapter 10—Oral diabetes medications..................................Page 121

This chapter focuses on pills. There are a ton of pills, but we'll break them down into broad categories for you. It looks at each pill's method of action, how to take them, and any side effects you need to look out for.

> The first pill—the sugar eater.. Page 121
> The second pill—the slave driver... Page 124
> The third pill—the anti-Pepto-Bismol................................... Page 126
> The fourth pill—complex and controversial .... Page 127
> The fifth pill—the new kid on the block .... Page 130
> Sometimes more is better .... Page 132

Chapter 11—Injectable diabetes medications................................. Page 133

Beyond pills are liquid medications that need to be injected. This chapter digs into these meds. We'll look at the method of action and side effects. The chapter also covers the various ways to deliver these meds into your body.

> Insulin—an oldie but goodie ....Page 136
> The first shot—rockin' around the clock ....Page 139
> The second shot—the race horse..Page 140
> MDI is not where you get your driver's license ....Page 141
> The third shot—the Model "T" ....Page 141
> Write your way to good health with an insulin pen................Page 143
> Shooting up! ....Page 144
> Insulin's dark side—hypos ....Page 147
> Two pens can sometimes be too many ....Page 148
> Higher tech than insulin pens—the insulin pump ....Page 150
> The fourth shot—the life saver...Page 152
> The fifth shot—a whole new kind of therapy from
>   lizard spit...Page 153

Chapter 12—Non-diabetes meds diabetics need .... Page 157

Of course you knew life wouldn't be as simple as just taking care of your blood sugar. There are a whole range of body systems at risk when you are diabetic. Many of these can be protected with yet more medications. From Aspirin to Zetia we'll cover them here. OK, we aren't really going to talk about Zetia, I just liked that whole A-to-Z thing….

> Eye of newt..Page 157
> All that you miss in your diet in one pill................................Page 158
> Lower your blood pressure and shield your kidneys..............Page 158
> Another ounce of prevention...Page 159

> "Poisons and medicine are oftentimes the same substance given with different intents."

Dr. Peter Mere Latham
19th-Century English Physician & Educator

Chapter 9—Doctors, medications, and you

Diabetes medication plans look like wedding cakes. We start with one layer, and if it doesn't quite do the job, we add a second layer. Of course, over time, the effectiveness of the medications begins to drop and the diabetes begins to advance. So we add another layer. And another.

I've actually seen older T-2s on as many as five diabetes meds. Which is insane. Very few folks, however, have the courage to pull out the bottom layer and see if the cake still stands. Our clinic does. Most of the time it makes no difference; the bottom layer has long since stopped being effective. But every once in a while we're wrong. We discontinue the bottom layer and damn if the patient's blood sugar doesn't go up. OK, no problem. We just restart it and the patient has to be content to do his or her part to support the pharmaceutical industry.

Two flavors, not thirty-one

D-meds come in pills, which we call *orals*; and liquids, which we call *injectables*. T-2s can, and will, use the entire range of the meds we're going to talk about in this chapter from top to bottom. Most pills will do no good whatsoever for T-1s and we get to play with the injectables from day one. The gestationally diabetic woman must use insulin only, one of the injectables. Virtually all of the orals can pass on to the fetus, and none of us want that. T-3s generally require only Advil or Tylenol and probably an anti-depressant or maybe high blood pressure pills. OK, I'm joking here folks. But have you got any idea how hard it is to live with *us*?

Diabetes drugs are widely misunderstood both by patients who take them and doctors who prescribe them. I know some pretty smart people who were given diabetes pills and thought that *that* took care of it.

And why not? We take our high blood pressure pills and our blood pressure ceases to be an issue, right? We take our cholesterol pills and our cholesterol ceases to be an issue, right? We take our thyroid pills and our thyroid ceases to be an issue, right? Shouldn't a diabetes pill fix the diabetes? Well of course not, but you can see why someone might think so.

Your partner not your boss

Next I need to tell you a couple of things about doctors. First let me state that I ***love*** doctors. They impress the hell out of me time and time again. The amount of assorted information they store in their heads, especially the general practice docs, just blows me away. If I knew even 5% of what my boss knows, I'm convinced my head would explode.

I've got it easy in my little nook of the medical profession. I really only need to know about one thing. It is an extraordinarily small "scope of practice" when compared to all that there is going on in the universe of medicine. Diabetes is my life—at work full time for years, and at home full time for many more years. It fills my study, my play, my days and my nights. I don't have a formal degree in diabetes, but I know it inside-and-out and backwards-and-forwards. I hate even to think about what percentage of my time is spent on diabetes.

But I'm told that most MDs only get two weeks of education on diabetes at med school. So in four years of school, a physician has only spent 0.0096% of his or her time on diabetes.

Don't forget that the vast majority of diabetes in our country is treated by family doctors, not specialists. In addition, most of these practices have neither a diabetes educator nor a nutritionist.

To top all of that off, how long does your doctor get to spend with you in a visit? The national average is just under ten minutes. Half that time will be spent typing frantically into a computer terminal or laptop to document the visit properly to keep the insurance companies and lawyers at bay.

By comparison, my standard visit with a patient is a full hour and I'm free to schedule much longer if I feel it is indicated.

Doctors are magnificent, extraordinary people who are working in possibly the worst conditions known to mankind. I admire them, but I don't envy them. Doctors absolutely have your best interests at heart, but you must understand your meds yourself.

Remember, *diabetes is a self-managed disease.* When you are on a medication you must understand how it works, how to take it, and what its possible side effects are. If you encounter any trouble along the way, do NOT be afraid to query your doc about it.

Most docs like thinking patients. If you happen to have one of the few who thinks he's God maybe it's time to shop for another. Your doctor is your partner, not your boss. Unless you work at a health center like I do. Then your boss is a doctor, which is still different from your doctor being your boss.

So on to the meds these noble, harassed, overworked men and women prescribe for you. Actually the first medication isn't a medication at all. It's a therapy.

The word "die" is part of diet

The old-school standard, when first diagnosing a patient with T-2 diabetes, is to prescribe *diet and exercise*. Sometimes you'd also be instructed to avoid stress. Oh, and stop smoking and not a drop of alcohol. Yeah. Right. I'll get right on that.

I even used to try framing the conversation in terms of, *OK we need to talk about nutrition and activity patterns.* My patients would get loooooooooooong faces. "You mean diet and exercise, don't you?"

Diet and exercise are dirty words.

The theory behind D&E is not completely without merit. Assuming your blood sugar is not at a life-threatening level (which it commonly is at diagnosis), changing your eating and activity patterns can cause you to lose weight. This weight loss can cause a T-2's insulin resistance to drop. That in turn *may* give the pancreas a chance to catch up. The diabetes can go into "remission" as long as the patient stays young and healthy. I used some cancer terminology intentionally here, even though it is not medically correct. I think if you have beaten back your diabetes with diet and exercise you really need to think of yourself like a cancer patient.

You never really beat cancer. We are not arrogant enough to think we can cure it. When we defeat an attack by chopping parts of your body off or out, zapping you with radiation, and poisoning you to within an inch of your life with chemo drugs, we only will go so far as to say the cancer has retreated. It is not necessarily gone. It is in remission. Maybe you never see it again. Maybe it is regrouping, rearming, getting ready for the next assault.

This is one reason cancer survivors are such fun people to be around. They've touched the face of death. They don't know how much more time they've been given. They often live each day to the fullest.

So here's the deal on diabetes "remission." If you succeed with diet and exercise you've only beat back the first assault. Diabetes is chronic—it never, ever goes away. It is progressive—it will always get worse. The risk in the diet and exercise approach as monotherapy is a lack of vigilance. It will work for a while, but it will ultimately fail.

That is why I say the theory is not completely without merit. It will work for a time. It will hold off the start of meds, which is good, as the clock is ticking on how long a given med will stay effective from the very first dose. And of course D&E will make you healthier and happier overall.

That said, I've pretty much kicked this therapy to the curb. Although I did once write a "prescription" for a bicycle….

D&E is damn hard for most folks to do or to maintain. In some cases impossible. If you ask people to do too much too early, you set them up for failure—and then everyone loses.

Bottom line: if you are dedicated enough and focused enough, you can make D&E therapy work for you. You can hold off T-2 for years, possibly a decade or more. But it is hard work. I know only two patients who succeeded with D&E, and then one of them got old enough that we had to start the meds anyway…

A kinder, gentler approach

My philosophy is that we should medicate people to a safe blood sugar level first, then introduce diet and exercise slowly, a step at a time. When the blood sugar is down again, people feel better. *Want to feel even better?* Now the door is open for change. My approach may be slower, but it works, and—most importantly—it is sustainable in the long run.

Of course, a T-1 can diet and exercise until the cows come home, but without insulin we die.

Chapter 10—Oral diabetes medications

o what do we have available to medicate your blood sugar to a safe level? Ah…we have a quiver full of arrows….

The first pill—the sugar eater

Meet the bottom layer of the wedding cake: metformin. This best-selling pill has been around for such a long time that it is now on the Wal-Mart $4 drug list. Metformin (part of a class of drugs called *biguanides*) is the generic name. It is also known under the Bristol-Myers Squib brand name of Glucophage, which is Latin for sugar-eater. If you take the less common Riomet, you are also taking metformin. Metformin is the most common starting point for oral drug therapy. In fact, the latest practice guidelines from the American Diabetes Association now suggest starting metformin at the time of diagnosis, *along* with diet and exercise.

Metformin does a couple of things, but its primary effectiveness is in addressing Leaky Liver Syndrome. The metformin holds back the constant drip of sugar from T-2's livers while they sleep. As this is often one of the early issues in T-2s, it makes metformin an ideal starting point.

Metformin also helps to a small degree with the absorption of carbs in the intestines, which can also help lower blood sugar spikes after eating. Because of this, metformin is commonly taken with meals.

Mets come in various sizes, typically 500, 850, and 1,000mg. Generally speaking you need to be on at least 1500mg per day to see any results, and the max daily dose is 2500mg. Metformin can cause upset stomach when first started, so it is often started in sub-effective doses of 500mg a day for two weeks to a month to get the body used to the med.

Metformin is a weight neutral drug, meaning it neither causes you to gain weight nor to lose weight.

For the most part, metformin is a harmless drug that plays well with others. It does have one quite rare side effect that you need to know about. Very, very, very rarely it causes a condition called *lactic acidosis,* a distant cousin of the T-1 diabetic coma.

Symptoms could include muscle pain or cramping, abdominal pain, nausea, vomiting, hyperventilation, reduced blood pressure, lethargy. The reason that this matters is that, although very rare, once it hits, it is fatal 50% of the time. Yikes! If you start on metformin and see these symptoms, don't even call your doctor, get the hell to the Emergency Room. You need serious medical intervention to save your life.

Now it is worth mentioning that metformin is contraindicated (medical word for a really, really, *really* bad idea) in patients who have reduced kidney function or liver disease. Accordingly, it is a tremendously bad idea to put an alcoholic on metformin.

So tell your doctor if you are a boozer. One of our standard questions when triaging patients at the clinic is to ask if they drink. Most folks tell me they are light drinkers. Where I came from originally, drinking light meant a glass of red wine with dinner once or twice per month. I innocently checked "light drinker" on the form for months until a "light drinker," who smelled pickled to me, told me he was a light drinker.

So how would you define light? I asked.

"Oh…. Twelve or fourteen beers," said the patient, perfectly calm, like he was commenting on what a nice day it was.

Per week? Asked little ol' innocent me.

"No. Per night," replied patient.

Holy crap. I'd die of alcohol poisoning if I drank 14 beers in a sitting!

Tell your doctor if you are a boozer.

If you need medical imaging (generally CAT scans or MRIs) that requires contrast dye, your doctor will have you stop taking the metformin before the imaging. Apparently met and intravenous contrast dyes do not play well together.

There is also an extended release version of met that is worth mentioning here. The medication is absorbed through the wall of the capsule, which then passes through the digestive tract intact, but empty. Patients tend to freak out when they think they are passing their medications.

The second pill—the slave driver

Next up comes a class of drugs called the *sulfonylureas*. The most common goes by the generic name of glipizide. The Pfizer brand name of glip is called Glucotrol. Other names in the same class of drugs include Amaryl, Diabinese, DiaBeta Micronase, and Glynase.
They all suck.

I guess I'd better qualify that. The purpose of this class of drugs is to stimulate the pancreas' insulin production. They grab the pancreas and squeeze it like a sponge to force out more insulin. That's one way to overcome insulin resistance: throw enough wood on the fire and you'll keep warm.

OK, here's the deal. I want you to picture the slave driver in the back of the Roman galley ship. The drums are beating. Thump…thump…thump…thump…The oars are creaking. The waves slap gently on the wooden hull.

Crack! The whip snaps. "Pull!"

Crack! "Pull!"

Crack! "Pull!"

Crack! "Pull!"

Crack! "Pull!"

Glipizide is the slave-driver drug. It stands over the poor enslaved pancreas with its whip causing the organ to secrete more insulin 24 hours a day, seven days per week, 365 days per year. This causes two very serious problems.

The first should be obvious. What happens to any machine, person, or tool that works non-stop? Oh, yeah, it breaks down. OK so the T-2's pancreas was already working overtime to try to overcome the insulin resistance, and now we're adding a night shift?

The second risk is hypoglycemia. These drugs have a 24-7-365 insulin-raising effect. What happens if you skip a meal? You can crash.

We've yanked an awful lot of people off glip. That said, I recommended that our medical director script it at least twice. In both cases for truck drivers who by Federal Law would have lost their commercial driver's licenses if they took insulin—which they really needed.

I always, always, always try to remember that our patients don't exist in a test tube. We humans are complex social creatures that exist in a spider web of family, society, economy, and other difficult realities.

Will the glip hurt these two men in the long run? Yes, I'm afraid so. Would losing their income right now hurt them more? Yes, definitely so.

Honorary members of this dark club include Starlix and Prandin. Technically they are in different drug classes, but they have a similar effect, with a slight twist: they have a short-lived action time. They are designed to stimulate the pancreas for only a short period of time.

The idea is that you take them with meals to give a boost of insulin production to cover the meal, then leave the pancreas alone the rest of the time. I rarely recommend either, but I'll leave them in place if someone comes to us using them and is in good control.

So I hate glip and its cousins. But I'm still glad to have that arrow in my quiver.

The third pill—the anti-Pepto-Bismol

Another class of oral drugs that is rarely used nowadays is the so called *Alpha-glucosidase Inhibitors*. Ouch. I'm sorry about all of these names. If it were up to me they'd all be in plain English like my online bank account password: CAT. Oh damn, I let the cat out of the bag now. I'll have to go change it to DOG.

The AGIs include the brand names Precose and Glyset. Their job is to slow the digestion of carbs to reduce glucose spikes. This sounds like a great idea on the surface, but the drugs have some nasty GI (gastro-intestinal) side effects that include "anal leakage."

Enough said about those, I guess. As we'll see in a bit, however, there is a new kid on the block that goes after digestion speed with awesome effect.

The fourth pill—complex and controversial

Now we come to one of the few orals that can be used by both T-1s and T-2s. The drugs called TZDs. Of course, that stands for the unpronounceable *thiazolidinediones*. TZDs include Actos and the much-maligned Avandia (more on that epic in a minute). TZDs are divinely complex drugs, and that may be part of the problem.

The theory is good—in fact, one of the best. TZDs are insulin sensitizers. Their job is to overcome the insulin resistance that is the main trouble in T-2 diabetes. Some T-1s also take TZDs too, because like the rest of the population, T-1s are becoming fatter and fatter and can also develop insulin resistance.

So TZDs make sure each insulin molecule leaving the pancreas has the house keys. Sounds great, right? Well TZDs work great! For controlling blood sugar, that is. The problem is that they make some folks swell up hugely, retaining fluid in their tissues. We call this *edema*. You usually see it first in the ankles and wrists, but the real issue is that if the tissue around the ankles and wrists swells up, so does the tissue around the heart, and that is… bad.

Other troubles include the fact that they can take from 4-6 weeks to start working. They are also incredibly hard on your liver. In a perfect world a blood test called an LFT (liver function test) should be done before starting a TZD and at least annually after that. But LFTs aren't cheap.

As a side note, virtually all medications are "filtered" by either the liver or the kidneys. I doubt anyone bothers to track it, but it would be ideal if we paid attention to how many liver-filtered meds you are on and how many kidney-filtered meds you are on, and make smart choices to avoid overworking either system.

About all you can do now is chat with your doctor about how your meds line up, and then choose whether to use Advil or Tylenol for your various aches and pains—as one is filtered by the liver and the other….

TZDs don't cause weight gain in the normal sense of the word. However, if you have the edema side effect mentioned above you could rapidly gain weight as the extra fluid in your tissues will show up on your bathroom scale as well as around your ankles and wrists.

So as promised, here is the story of the Avandia debacle. In a nutshell: at one time, Avandia was one of the most commonly prescribed D-meds in the world. As a blood sugar lowering agent I found it to be more effective than its competitor Actos. Then a study was published in the *New England Journal of Medicine* that suggested a possible link to a significantly increased number of heart attacks in Avandia users. The mass media caught wind of it and D-folks in droves stopped taking Avandia. Overnight. Many didn't even bother to call their doctors to tell them. The rest tried to call and got the message "all circuits are busy, please try your call later."

Is Avandia bad news? I don't know. Here's the problem: the study in question re-crunched data from previous studies in a controversial statistical technique called meta-analysis. Those previous studies, not really looking at heart stuff, made no attempt to collect coronary data. So here is the problem: we know heart attacks finish off most D-folk, and a study of D-folk finds a bunch on a certain med kick the bucket from heart attacks while taking that med. Hmmmmm....

Now more of the Avandia users kicked the bucket than those on other meds, but was the sample good? Could those patients have been ones that had already had five heart attacks? Maybe. Maybe not.

Other previously published clinical studies, some with very large numbers of patients, showed no difference in heart attack deaths between various D-therapies; including comparisons between the very-safe metformin and the TZDs.

Once the Avandia meta-analysis hit the evening news, the maker of Avandia could have handled the situation…hmmmm…how do I say this without getting my pants sued off? They could have handled it……better. Enough said.

At that point, however, it really didn't matter. Maybe the med is safe. Maybe the med is dangerous. But like I said, it didn't really matter. The patients were scared of it.

I sat down with our medical director and he decided to take all of our patients who used Avandia off the med. We decided to err on the side of caution, because it wasn't like we didn't have alternatives. Lots of wedding cake to go around.

But I do miss Avandia. It really did work. At least at knocking down blood sugar.

And based on the rationale that by the time most T-2s are dx'd pancreatic function is already reduced, some new practice guidelines urge starting a TZD as the first line of therapy along with diet and exercise.

Despite the problems with the TZDs, more are on the horizon, pending FDA approval.

The fifth pill—the new kid on the block

The last pill to talk about is the newest kid on the block and is part of a whole new class of drugs that looks at diabetes in a whole new way.

Remember when I told you that the tibia connects to the patella and the patella connects to the… That's right. Nothing in medicine is simple, because nothing in the human body is simple. Ergo, nothing in diabetes is simple either.

OK, we got that whole pancreas and insulin and insulin resistance thing down pat, right? Well, as you might expect, things aren't turning out to be that simple, after all.

That whole digestion, insulin, hormone thing has a larger cast of characters than we suspected a while back and the newest players on the stage are *incretins*.

OK, this whole incretin thing makes my head hurt, but here we go! The two new words you need to learn today are GLP-1 and DPP-4. Sorry, that's what we're stuck with. Bear with me here.

These two incretins have a symbiotic relationship. DPP-4's job is to stamp out GLP-1 when it finishes its job. GLP-1's job is to regulate the speed of digestion and to properly coordinate the telegraph between the stomach and the brain; in other words, the ability of the stomach to tell the brain when it is full so that you know you have eaten enough.

In T-2s, DPP-4 jumps the starting gate. It gets out too soon. It wipes out the GLP-1 before it can do its job properly. The net result is that with the GLP-1 out of the picture, the stomach dumps its contents too quickly into the intestines. The telegraph lines have also been cut by hostile natives; not only is the stomach now actually empty, the brain never got the signal that food arrived in the first place. Many T-2s are *always* hungry.

Meanwhile the intestines are overloaded and they are where most carbs are absorbed into the bloodstream. Lots of sugar hits the system. The blood sugar spikes. When your sugar is high, perversely, you get hungry, and on it goes….The first incretin medication that addressed this problem is an injectable, so we'll talk about it later. The second is a pill called Januvia.

Januvia is a DPP-4 inhibitor. So the job of this pill is to keep the DDP-4 at bay so the GLP-1 can do its job. On the surface it looks elegant and simple. In practice the jury is out. Seems to work extraordinarily well for some folks, not so well for others. The earlier on you are in your diabetes, the better it will probably work for you but the less likely your insurance will cover it.

Januvia is weight neutral.

And that, as of today, is the end of the approved orals for your blood sugar. But of course, we are facing a huge T-2 epidemic worldwide. There is a lot of money to be made on diabetes, and given that most people are needle-phobic, there will be a huge market for pills. I'm sure we will see dozens of new orals over the next decade. Some will be wonderful, some will be minimally useful, some may be dangerous. But we'll have many more arrows in our quiver.

Sometimes more is better

Wrapping up the chapter on orals I want to point out that there is a ton of clinical evidence that shows using any two drugs to attack diabetes is always more effective in both the short and long term, than using any one drug by itself. We call this combo-therapy vs. monotherapy. As most folks get sloppy about taking their pills as the volume of pills increases, there are a variety of poly-pills available that mix two kinds of diabetes orals into one capsule. Examples would include metformin and TZD in one pill or metformin and Januvia. Poly-pills do make your life easier and might replace two co-pays with one. The more cynical among us will point out that this approach also allows drug companies to take a generic pill, mix it with something else and sell it for more money. Bottom line for me is that if it helps people take all their meds, it is a good thing. *Ask your doctor if poly-pills are right for you.*

Chapter 11—Injectable diabetes medications

I still remember the scariest day of my life. Misdiagnosed as a T-2, my health was rapidly spiraling downhill out of control. My wonderful, modest, caring family doctor threw up his hands and checked his ego at the door. "I don't know what's going on with you, but we need to get you to a specialist," he told me. That process would take six weeks. To keep me alive until then, he put me on a 24-hour insulin.

"You need to take your shot in the stomach," he told me.

Picturing a huge needle piercing my skin, fat, muscle, and tearing straight into the organ of my stomach itself, a vision of horrible pain came to me. Wouldn't my stomach acid leak out? My face must have lost all color, because he quickly corrected himself: "Sorry, my brain suffers from being in Spanish half the time and English half the time. I meant to say 'abdomen.'"

That didn't sound a whole lot more comforting to me. Much later I'd learn that the skin around your belly button is more devoid of nerve endings than pretty much anywhere else on your body. Shots are taken there because that is the area where they will hurt the least.

My family doctor had neither the time nor staff for training patients how to take shots. He sent me home with two prescriptions. One for insulin. One for syringes. No instructions beyond, "You're a smart guy, you'll figure it out."

At home that night I tore open the bag of syringes and laid one on the table. I took the insulin vial from its cardboard box. It was time to give myself my first shot.

I was on my own for this ordeal. My wife Deb and my little son Rio, as unused to being T-3s as I was unused to being diabetic, were nowhere to be found. They're probably hiding somewhere in the back of the house, I thought to myself grimly.

I consulted the various sheets of paper the pharmacy sent home with me and then unscrewed the orange cap at the base of the syringe. I pulled the plunger back to pull air into the tube. I pried the purple cap off of the tall, thin vial of insulin. Under the cap was a rubber membrane.

I slid the needle through it, and then held the vial upside down, the syringe sticking out the bottom. I injected the air into the vial, then pulled the plunger back down again. Ice-clear liquid tumbled into the barrel of the syringe.

I don't recall my starting dose, but I pulled down more than I needed and removed the syringe from the vial. Holding the syringe vertically, I slowly pushed the plunger upwards. First air escaped, then a narrow stream of insulin spurted into the air. The faint smell of Band-Aids reached my nostrils, the scent of insulin.

The syringe was ready. It was time. I hesitated. For a *looooooooooooooong* time.

Sticking a needle into your skin is the most unnatural act known to mankind. It takes incredible will power and courage to do it the first time.

I gently rested the needle against my skin and gathered up my courage. And then…. And then….

And then I pulled the needle away and started to hyperventilate. *Holy shit! And I have to do this for six weeks? Maybe longer? I can't do this!*

So I pulled myself together again and rested the needle against my bare skin. And then…. And then…

And then I pulled the needle away. *Crap! I'm such a chicken shit!*

And then, closing my eyes and holding my breath, I drove the needle into my stomach like a disgraced samurai committing hara-kiri… and….

I felt nothing. Nothing at all. No pain…..No…. nothing.

I opened my eyes and I let my breath out. Then I slowly injected the clear fluid. I pulled the needle out and looked at it.

Well, maybe that sucker isn't so big after all… The needle that looked like a fencing foil 60 seconds ago now looked more like a human eyelash.

The average T-1 will take at least 100,000 shots in his or her lifetime, but none of us can ever forget that first shot.

That's why if you are my patient your first shot will take place in my office; you with real insulin, me with saline. We do it together. In a loving, supportive environment. And it is no big deal.

After days, weeks, months, maybe years of fear, patients all say the same thing: "Hey! That wasn't so bad! The finger sticks hurt worse!"

And it is true. I promise you. The finger sticks that you are used to hurt ten times more than the shot. The shot is no big fucking deal at all.

Insulin—an oldie but goodie

A hormone called *insulin* is the oldest of the diabetes injectables, and it now comes in a variety of flavors.

Prior to the 1920s no one in the medical world even knew what insulin was. In a great many ways insulin was as ahead-of-its-time as Leonardo da Vinci was ahead of his time.

A few cold-hearted bastards have even stated regret that the treatment was discovered at all. They feel the availability of a *treatment* has reduced the pressing need for a *cure*.

As a person who lives, breathes, is a husband and a father; I gotta say I'd rather be kept alive by a *treatment* than be dead. Of course I've also been cynical enough to tell people that I believe that diabetes has been cured at least seven times and that each time the big drug companies have shot the researcher in the head, buried his body in a cornfield, and burned his research. There is a lot more money to be made in treatments than in cures.

That said, we live longer (which allows us to spend more) and better lives with every year and every advance in insulin.

The original insulins were made by mashing up animal pancreases and distilling the insulin "juice" out of them. For many years beef and pork insulin were the rule.

Now we have artificial insulin. Its DNA is similar to human insulin, but it is…well, more or less synthetic. It has, in some cases, been altered to act a little differently than the real stuff. Native insulin is mainlined into the body's blood vessels by the pancreas but we shoot our magic DNA-modified insulin "subQ," into the fat layer between the skin and the muscle.

We T-1s take insulin to replace what we lack. You T-2s are more complex and your mileage may differ. Some T-2s have worn out their pancreases. After years of fighting insulin resistance the pancreas gives up the ghost. In some cases the pancreas sputters along still producing some insulin. In other cases, like with T-1s, it ceases to produce any at all. In either case the T-2 patient now needs insulin. This will happen to all T-2s in the fullness of time.

In the other case, the T-2's pancreas is working triple time and doing a damn fine job; but it is no use. The insulin resistance is so severe it cannot be overcome naturally. If TZDs won't work we add supplemental insulin. Just like the overworked pancreas trying to keep up, we are overwhelming the insulin resistance with so much insulin that the resistance just doesn't stand a chance.

Insulin is not weight neutral, and the reasons for this are hotly contended. A good deal of clinical data shows that patients who are put on insulin, on the whole, gain weight. No one argues that fact, but the mechanism of that weight gain is contested; some folks think the medication causes weight gain while others feel a change in patient behavior is to blame. Still another possibility is linked to improved control. More on that in a second.

To make some oral meds work, you need to be more careful about moderating your diet. In theory, once you are on insulin you can eat any damn thing you want, so long as you *bolus* (taking a dose of insulin) properly for it. Cheesecake? Sure. Twinkies? Why not? Just look up the carbs and take a big enough shot. Some experts believe this new-found dietary freedom is what causes the weight gain.

The improved control theory, on the other hand, is based on the fact that when your BGLs are very high your body is desperate to get the sugar out. The best way for the body to do that is through urine. Folks with high BGLs pee all the time, some getting up 3, 4, 6 times per night. A ton of calories get dumped into the urine with the sugar. Once supplemental insulin is added the BGLs drop and the extra calories go to the waistline instead of into the toilet.

Now I *lost* a ton of weight when I went *on* insulin. The exact opposite of what the clinical data shows happens to most people, so for a long time I thought the weight gain associated with insulin was linked to behavior. Now I'm not so sure. I've seen patients who are very careful about what they eat gain weight. So for now, I'm content to let it be one of those your-mileage-may-vary mysteries that we just need to be alert to.

In today's world we have three broad types of insulin: basal, fast acting, and…other.

The first shot—rockin' around the clock

Let's start with basal insulin, not because it is the oldest, but because it is the one T-2s will need to get to know before the others. There are two basal insulins: Lantus and Levemir.

Although they differ chemically, the net result is the same: this is a once a day shot for most people. The effect of the insulin lasts for approximately 24 hours. Lantus is the older of the two. Each little super-micro drip of the Lantus insulin is wrapped in bubble wrap. Once in your body, the bubble wrap begins to dissolve, releasing the insulin into your system a little at a time.

Levemir acts the same way, except that it uses the black magic of molecular chemistry rather than bubble wrap. Depending on dosing, we often find that the Levemir gives patients a "flatter" BGL profile than Lantus does; a between-meal blood sugar graph of a Lantus shooter looks like a washboard road. Levemir drivers are on the Autobahn; but in many folks it won't last the full 24-hours, requiring two shots per day.

That said, they are both damn good drugs. Although intended in both cases for once-a-day dosing, we'll often have patients take both a bedtime and morning shot. By making one dose larger than the other we can play games with the dosing that can help us give our patients more control.

Most T-2s start with basal insulin. It will "lower the bar" for the whole day. Every T-1 needs basal to keep BGLs in target between meals and overnight.

The second shot—the race horse

Fast-acting insulins currently come in three varieties: Humalog, NovoLog, and Apidra. All three are made by different manufacturers, but are very similar. Certain individuals will often find that one or the other works better for them, but they are to a very large degree interchangeable.

After injection, fast-acting insulins peak in two hours, and are gone from your system in 4-6 hours in most folks. They are designed to be taken with meals to knock down the excursion and help the body metabolize the carbs from the meal.

This is one reason why the two-hour-after-you-eat blood sugar check is so important. You are halfway through the insulin's action curve. If you are at…oh…say 118, should you be happy? Hell no! You've got two hours of insulin left. You're gonna crash!

MDI is not where you get your driver's license

Virtually all T-1s and some T-2s take both basal and fast-acting insulin. This is called MDI (for multiple daily injection) or Basal/Bolus therapy. *Bolus* is a medical and patient slang term for an injection of fast-acting insulin taken with a meal.

I use MDI to keep myself healthy.

One important note for you fellow T-1s: basal is not a foundation; in fact, it is shifting sand under your feet. Your basal should be about half of your daily insulin. The misunderstood bummer is that this is not a fixed amount at all. If you have a really, really, really high carb day—you went to China Star's all-you-can-eat buffet and then to Cold Stone Creamery—you will need more basal. When you have low-carb yogurt for breakfast, a salad for lunch, and salmon and green beans for dinner; you need less basal.

Many T-1s try to muddle through with a set basal rate. This will work if your day-to-day carb intake is stable; otherwise you need to adjust on the fly.

The third shot—the Model "T"

The "other" category includes stone tools and bear skins, the now rarely used "mix" insulins, and another old-school insulin called NPH. While all modern insulins are clear, NPH is a milky, thick-looking liquid. It was the first generation of bubble-wrapped insulin, with a duration of action in the 8-12 hour zone. Before modern basals it was used to keep us T-1s alive overnight without having to wake up every four hours and take a shot.

Even within a single patient, NPH is somewhat....erratic… in its action. It is rarely used except by uninsured folks who earn just a little too much to qualify for patient assistance programs. The only thing NPH has going for it, compared to more modern insulins, is its price.

Several insulin companies make different "mix" insulins. These combine the mid-range NPH and similar insulins with a fast-acting insulin. The idea is to reduce the number of shots necessary in an MDI-style therapy.

The problem is caused by how the shots can overlap. Depending on the number and timing of shots, it is easy to accidentally "stack" the actions of the two types of insulin, resulting in *hypoglycemia,* or low blood sugar. Our clinic has only one patient still on mix and we've taken dozens off so they won't pass out, drive off the road and hit trees.

If you are the type of person who eats right on schedule and lives on a rigid schedule every day, mix is probably safe enough. It is good for inflexible old men. And women.

Write your way to good health with an insulin pen

In the old days insulin only came in vials. In the really old days you had to sharpen your needles on a whetstone and boil the glass syringes on top of the stove!

Vials are still around, as are disposable one-shot syringes, but the state of the art is the insulin pen. The disposable variety is the most common: a plastic tube about the size and shape of a fountain pen. It comes preloaded (usually with 300 units of joy juice) and is ready to use. You just screw on a pen needle, dial up your dose on a wheel at the bottom and shoot. What could be easier?

There are also metal pens that take disposable refill cartridges. Some use half-unit dosing for insulin-sensitive types and kiddos; and at least one model has a memory so you can check mid-meal to see if you remembered to take your insulin (hey, you do it every meal, every day…over time one shot is so much like another that all of us "forget" to dose now and again).

I think insulin pens are wonderful and take a lot of the hassle out of the daily grind of diabetes.

Shooting up!

While we are on insulin, so to speak, let's touch on the subject of injection technique.

Starting at the business end of the pen, we have the disposable pen needle. One pen might use many needles before it is empty.

The pen needle, before it is used, has a paper back. It looks kinda like a miniature Mercury space capsule. The paper backing has a tab. Pull off the tab and throw it away. Screw the space capsule onto the pen. Now it's really starting to look like a rocket ship!

Screwing the pen needle on is a lot like screwing on the caps on your car's tires after filling them with air. Once it is on, pull the milky white plastic part off. Yep, turns out the capsule was just a sterile cover. If you have a cat, throw this piece on the floor because cats just love playing with them. If you don't have a cat, just throw this part in the trash. You don't need it anymore.

Now you'll see a pencil lead-like piece of plastic. It might be white, it might be purple, depending on the brand and size of the needle. That's the needle cover. Pull it off carefully, being sure not to bend it to either side. Now you'll see a ridiculously small needle.

No fear.

Spin the dial on your pen to "1" or "2" and do what we call an "air shot." Make sure you get a little squirt of insulin or a drop at the tip of the needle. Some more cynical diabetics claim this is a way to make all of us collectively waste, and therefore buy, thousands of gallons of insulin more per year than we can use.

True….but you don't want air in your needle. It won't harm you—this isn't a shot you take in a vein—but it can throw off your dose.

Now, dial up your dose. Hold the pen perpendicular to your skin. Slide it in. Inject. Count ten seconds in your head…

One-thousand-one, one-thousand-two, one-thousand-three, one-thousand-four, one-thousand-five, one-thousand-six, one-thousand-seven, one-thousand-eight, one-thousand-nine, one-thousand-ten.

You are done.

Pull the needle out of your body and replace the little cap, being careful not to bend the needle.

Most D-folk who use pens like the "homicidal maniac" hold; gripping the pen with one hand, thumb on the base like you are lunging at someone with a knife held overhead. Of course you need to turn it on yourself. You slip the needle in and then press the button with your thumb.

You don't need to use alcohol pads anymore. You can even shoot through your clothes if you want to. Don't get a favorite spot. If you always inject in the same spot you'll build up scar tissue which can give you nasty little bumps on your sexy flat stomach and make it impossible for the insulin to diffuse into your tissues in a reliable, repeatable manner.

If, like most of us, you shoot in the "stomach," keep two inches away from your belly button. You can also use your thigh or upper arm. The upper arm is in vogue with the T-1 kids. I tried it once 'cause it looks so cool the way they calmly whip out their pens and elegantly inject into their arms. But for me it hurt like hell.

The folks that make pen needles will tell you to use a fresh one each time you inject. The fact is you may or may not be able to use it again. It depends on how thick your hide is.

I can use a needle for about a week before it gets dull. I know one diabetic who can go a month. Some of my patients can only use a needle two or three times. How do you know when it is dull? When it hurts to take a shot.

You do not need to keep modern insulin, basal or fast-acting, in the fridge. At least not the pen you are using. If your pharmacy has given you five pens for the month, keep the spares with your lettuce, cucumbers, and milk, but the pen you are using can stay at room temperature.

Once the pen is breached with its first needle the clock is ticking. The pen now has an official life of 30 days and a realistic life of 45 days regardless of how much you use. Keeping it in the fridge will not extend its life, but will only make your shots hurt like hell. Most bodies don't like cold fluids injected into them.

Some T-2s use very large quantities of basal insulin; 60, 80, even 120 units a day and more. There is no ceiling to insulin. You take as much as you need to get the job done. There is even a special 5x strength fast-acting called U-500 for insulin-resistant folks.

You might be given instructions to self-titrate: increasing your insulin on your own by 5 or ten units per day until you reach your target blood glucose. Remember self management?

Insulin's dark side—hypos

Other than the controversial weight-gain issue, insulin generally plays well with other meds, does not screw up your liver or your kidneys and seems to have only one major side effect. If you take too much your blood sugar will go too low.

Insulin and blood glucose exist in a diametrically opposed symbiotic relationship. They are poison and antidote to each other. Too much sugar? Take insulin. Too much insulin? Take sugar.

Remember that chaotic world we all live in? So you go to your favorite restaurant. But today, although you don't know it, Bill, the regular cook, didn't make it to work. His wife left him for his father and he is at a bar getting drunk. Hey, it could happen. Joe is filling in. *He* makes your favorite recipe different than Bill does. You take your usual insulin and three hours later it feels like the cables just broke on the elevator. Your hands are shaking. Your face sweating. And you find yourself frantically trying to pull out your medical alert necklace so the cops won't taser you.

The once- or twice-a-month hypo is the cost of doing business on insulin. That is why you should **always** carry your meter with you. **Always** wear your alert jewelry. **Always** carry some emergency sugar (glucose tabs, hard candy, or one of those little 4 oz bottles of liquid glucose).

Two pens can sometimes be too many

Most T-2s use much less fast-acting than basal (for T-1s it is 50-50); and when you use both there is always the risk of picking up the wrong pen and taking the wrong kind of insulin. I remember the first time this happened to one of our patients. My cell phone rang at a little after nine at night:

"Sorry to bug you at home, but I really fucked up."

How so?

"I mixed up my pens."

In a flash I knew what had happened. *You just took fast-acting instead of basal?*

"Yeah. I'm scared shitless."

No fear. We can fix this. How many units did you take?

"Seventeen. Of NovoLog. I can't fucking believe I did that."

This guy is pretty insulin-sensitive. Seventeen units is more fast-acting than he usually takes in the better part of a week. *Bygones. Shit happens. Don't worry about it. Tell me what you've got to eat in the house that's sweet.*

He had a few glucose tabs, a pint of Ben and Jerry's chocolate ice cream and granular sugar for his hummingbird feeder. No juice, soda, honey. *OK, start eating the ice cream... No, all of it...* I don't let any fear creep into my voice, but I know this is damn serious. I need to get about 300 carbs into my guy to soak up the insulin.

He tells me the package of sugar he has for the hummers reports four carbs per teaspoon. I call up the recipe math website on my laptop. *OK.* Three teaspoons in a tablespoon…so 12 carbs per tablespoon…four tablespoons in a quarter cup….so 48 carbs in a quarter cup….four quarters makes a cup…so a full cup of sugar has 192 carbs.

I want you to mix a cup of sugar into four cups of water and drink it down. I chose 4 cups to make it quick and easy to get the sugar into solution. I stay on the phone while he mixes the concoction and drinks it down.

"It's pretty nasty," he reports.

He survived just fine. Other diabetics have not been so lucky. I've noticed recently that the identical pens that hold the various juices now have large colorful labels rather than the little colored bands they used to have. I'd still love to see fast-acting fluid colored red instead of clear. Stop, Look, Listen. Think before you shoot.

Higher tech than insulin pens—the insulin pump

I want to touch quickly on a really cool medical device available to most T-1s and some T-2s as an alternative to the insulin pens and MDI shots. It is called the *insulin pump*. Most pumps are high-tech pager-sized devices that have a small reservoir of fast-acting insulin in them.

The pump connects to the diabetic by a thin plastic hose. (There is one pump with a different design where the insulin is held in a "pod" taped to your body so it does not need the hose.)

You wear something called an *infusion set*, which is basically a port for the insulin to get into your body. Every three or four days you shoot one of these into your body. It has a guide needle that comes out and only leaves a tiny tube in you called a *cannula*. It is basically one shot every three days instead of 5-8 shots per day for the typical MDI diabetic.

The pump holds only fast-acting insulin, and your basal needs are covered by an adjustable constant drip of insulin. The advantage is obvious in that you can match the basal "pattern" to the unique and changing needs of your body more precisely than you can with one or two long-acting insulin shots per day.

Meal boli are covered with a press of a button. Some pumps even do the math for you if you just tell the pump how many carbs the meal has, and some even help you figure *that* out.

Some diabetics swear by them, some don't like to be tethered. Many people will argue that you will have better control with a pump. Well….

OK, I can speak to this with some authority, as I started out with MDI, then got a pump. I've even used three of the most common brands of pumps. Then our insurance changed at the clinic and I could no longer afford to pump and had to go back to MDI. I was pretty hot under the collar for a while…*grumble, grumble…medical professional not being able to afford the* **standard** *of care…grumble, grumble…*

But it actually ended up being a good thing. It got me back in the trenches with my patients and taught me the fundamental truth about pumps and MDI: it is possible to have crappy control on either shots or pumps. It is also possible to have sublime control on either pumps or shots.

For many, pumps do make it easier to keep their sugar in control, and that's a good thing. But it is important to remember that the pump only replaces your pancreas, not your brain. You still have to think. This is a fancy, elegant insulin delivery device—not an automatic pancreas.

The fourth shot—the life saver

All of you that use fast-acting insulin and have a T-3 that loves you should have a Glucagon Emergency Kit. Made by both Novo Nordisk and Ely Lilly (the only difference is one is in a red plastic case, the other orange), the kits contain a powdered hormone and a syringe of saline. If you get so low you pass out—it can and does happen—no kidding this time; your T-3 can save your life by shooting this into you. It will cause the liver to dump all the stored glucose it has into your body, bringing you back from the other side.

To use the kit, your T-3 needs to keep his or her head. They need to inject the water into the vial, mix it around, then draw it in again, before shooting you. The glucagon is very unstable and short lived, that's why the crazy process. No epi-pens for us! Many T-3s worry about hurting their loved one with the needle if they inject "wrong." Hey, we're unconscious at this point, we won't feel a thing.

Tell your T-3 to turn you on your side (you'll most likely throw up) and then call 911. Unless you've collapsed on an expensive oriental rug in which case the procedure is: shoot, drag, turn, call. *Even if you feel OK when you come out of it, you still need to go to the hospital.* Like earthquakes, bad hypos sometimes have after-shocks and now your liver has nothing left to give.

Like the old-fashioned fire drill in grade school, using the kit is something the two of you should practice. Do "dry" runs, simulating the water injection, powder mixing, etc. Once you have an expired kit, have your T-3 go through the entire process, injecting an orange in the final step. Don't eat the orange. Speaking of expired kits, check your hypo kit's expiration date when you change your smoke detector batteries. You *do* change your smoke detector batteries, don't you?

The fifth shot—a whole new kind of therapy from lizard spit

The last injectable is in the same class as the last of the orals we talked about: incretins. In this case we have a wonder-drug called Byetta, a drug for T-2s only. Remember the DPP-4 and GLP-1 dance? The pill held back the DPP-4. Byetta works the other way around, giving you extra GLP-1 (well, technically a synthetic version called a mimetic), overwhelming the DPP-4 in the same way insulin shots overwhelm insulin resistance. People love the fact that Byetta was developed from studying Gila Monster saliva. I've had patients walk into my office and announce, "I want that lizard spit drug!"

Like insulin, it comes in a pen. Like metformin, you need to start with a smaller dose. Like nothing else in the arsenal, you lose a ton of weight.

What? Did that wake you up? Yep, the major side effect for most folks on this med is huge weight loss. I've seen folks shed 30 pounds on this in six weeks!

It is taken twice per day before the major meals. It slows the stomach down and repairs the telegraph wires between the stomach and the brain that the natives cut. Patients feel fuller faster. One very, very, very, obese woman told me she'd felt like she was starving for her entire life—until she took Byetta. "It took a monkey off my back," she told me.

This drug can actually restore first-phase insulin response in some patients. If we lived in a *just* world, this would be the medication of first resort when a patient is newly diagnosed.

But we live in a crappy world and most insurance plans require a patient to "fail" at cheaper therapies for various periods of time before they will approve Byetta.

Byetta, nationwide, makes a lot of folks very sick to their stomachs when they first start it. We've had very little trouble at our clinic and I think it's our approach. We spend a lot of time emphasizing how you are *not* going to need to eat as much as you used to. We'll make you buy smaller plates. Eat tiny servings, wait, assess whether or not you are still hungry, then eat more if indicated.

Some T-2s find they only eat 10% of what they used to. But they feel full, energetic, and happy (so in reality they were overeating by 90%). The drug doesn't really cause you to lose weight. It causes you to eat what you need, and that's what causes the weight loss. The trick to succeeding with Byetta is to truly tune in to what your body is telling you. We eat by habit. If you always eat half the pizza you will always eat half the pizza—whether you need it or not. If you always eat the whole pizza, you'll always eat the whole pizza—whether you need it or not.

You need to break from habit. Listen to your stomach. Eat what you need.

One last wonderful thing about Byetta is that its duration of action is linked to your glucose level. Once you are low enough, it simply shuts off. Kinda like automatic insulin, how cool is that?

There have been a limited number of cases of *pancreatitis* (a painful and sometimes dangerous inflammation of the pancreas) in Byetta users that probably got more media attention than the number of cases justified. The maker has added a new warning to the box and research continues; but at this point there is really no evidence to suggest that the attacks were caused by the medication.

Byetta has several competitors pending FDA approval as of this writing; and I think various incretin therapies are the wave of the future.

For T-1s Byetta also has a cousin named Symlin. Although not really the same on a bio-chemical level, the usage and effect is very similar. The only thing to be aware of is that you still need to take your insulin, but you will need less, possibly half the amount you used before.

On all meds, both oral and injectable: if your blood sugars are still above target you need more of your current medication or the addition of a new layer of the wedding cake. *Ask your doctor if more wedding cake is right for you.*

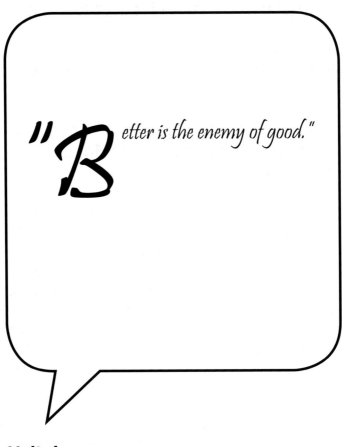

"Better is the enemy of good."

Voltaire
Writer & Philospher

Chapter 12—Non-diabetes meds diabetics need to take, and why

Other than the meds you take for blood sugar, there are four more pills that all D-folk should take every day for overall health: a baby aspirin, a multi-vitamin, an ACE and statin.

Eye of newt, toe of frog, wool of bat, tongue of dog... and willow bark. Seriously. At least about the willow bark.

But I'm not a baby! you say. OK, here's the deal: there is a ton of clinical research that shows aspirin therapy hugely reduces the risk of both heart attack and stroke. As it is heart attacks that do in most D-folk, 81 milligrams of prevention is worth a pound of cure. The "baby" aspirin are very small low-dose pills, more appropriate for a small amount in your body, and reducing the risk of blood clots, than for treating headaches. It is a small enough dose that most people won't get upset stomach with a baby aspirin. If you have a super-delicate stomach you can find a *buffered* baby aspirin. Buffered pills have a coating that holds them together until they pass through the stomach and into the intestines.

Unless you have an allergy to aspirin or are on a medication that would contraindicate its use, you should really do this! Hey, but don't be a bone head, ask your primary care provider first!

All that you miss in your diet in one pill

As to the multi-vitamin, I'm not sure you'll actually see this in any formal practice guidelines, so this might just be one of my own pet peeves. The American diet is horrible. We really don't eat healthy enough, even those of us who try. I believe a daily multi fills in the gaps between what we eat and what our bodies need. Personally, even though I'm not totally gray, I use Centrum Silver. It's formulated for older folks, but I figure as a person with a progressive chronic illness I'm an honorary senior citizen. There are a million multis out there, both brand-name and store-name. There is even one that is supposed to be formulated especially for diabetics. If you compare the looooooong list of what they all have in them, it is pretty much the same. Choose something you like the price and sound of and add it to your daily pillbox.

Lower your blood pressure and shield your kidneys

An ACE (a.k.a. ACE Inhibitor) is actually a high blood pressure pill. As you might have guessed, ACE stands for Angiotensin-Converting Enzyme. Research shows that in addition to lowering blood pressure ACEs have a kidney-shielding effect. Taking an ACE can protect your kidneys from your blood sugar to some degree. It used to be that an ACE was added once a diabetic starting spilling microalbumin in his or her urine, the first sign of kidney damage. Recently the *why jack around, let's be proactive* approach has taken hold and the practice guidelines suggest putting all D-folk, except pregnant females, on ACEs before the horse has left the barn.

If your blood pressure is also high you can kill two birds with one stone. If your blood pressure is really, really high then the ACE can be part of the solution. If your blood pressure is just peachy-keen you can still take a low-dose ACE without suffering from hypotension, or low blood pressure.

Another ounce of prevention

This same rationale has led to the somewhat new recommendation to add a statin to your daily lineup. Statins are cholesterol drugs. The new let's-close-the-barn-door-before-the-horse-leaves approach advocates adding a low-dose statin before your cholesterol gets high. I actually think that this is a hell of a good idea because cholesterol is shown to have a significant relationship to heart attacks and we all know what kills most diabetics, right? Statins include the famous Lipitor, as well as Mevacor, Crestor, and Zocor among others. One thing to remember with statins is that you need to give up your grapefruit habit. For bio-chemical reasons beyond me, grapefruit and statins don't play well together—sometimes causing the statin to over-perform and sometimes to under-perform, even in the same patient.

No regular soda. No sugar in your coffee. No grapefruit. Welcome to diabetes. You can still have all the steak you want, small amounts of popcorn, an occasional beer, and sex.

Or maybe not.

> "Diabetes is like being expected to play the piano with one hand wile juggling items with another hand, all while balancing iwth deftness and dexterity on a tight rope."

Marlene Less, Diabetic (type unknown)
Most frequently quoted diabetic online

Section 5—The Real World

Chapter 13—Sex, drugs, and rock & roll ....Page 163

In this chapter we get to talk about sex, or at least how diabetes can affect it. It also looks at other "vices" such as drugs that didn't come from your doctor, drinking, and smoking. It covers the cost of diabetes and stress. And we'll talk about your family and how they affect your diabetes. It wraps up with how the real world will collide with our best efforts to control our diabetes, and what to do about it.

> Dollars and sense.. Page 164
> Alcohol and diabetes .... Page 165
> Drugs, not the kind you get a prescription for....................... Page 167
> Diabetes and stress .... Page 168
> Taking a vacation from your diabetes .... Page 168
> Smoking .... Page 170
> High blood pressure and other things that cause trouble........ Page 173
> La Familia .... Page 174
> Twinkies and corn chips, a world of temptation .... Page 177

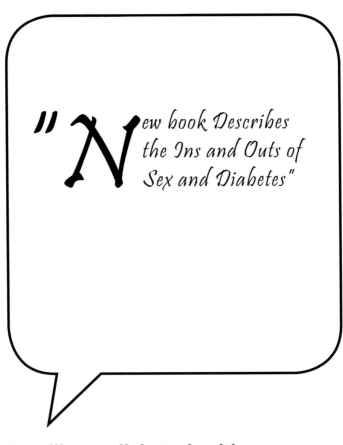

"*New book Describes the Ins and Outs of Sex and Diabetes*"

Headline at diabeteshealth.com
(no kidding)

Chapter 13—Sex, drugs, and rock & roll

So let's talk about sex. Ummm, OK, remember all those distal capillaries we were talking about in the hands, feet, eyes, and kidneys? Well there is one other spot on the human body, specifically on a man's body, where there are quite a few capillaries that I neglected to talk about earlier. Below his waist. Above his knees. On his anterior side. I think everyone is with me here, but just in case, I'll blurt it right out: *a man's penis is chock-full of capillaries.*

So, guys, here's the bad news: fully half (50%) of men with diabetes suffer from erectile dysfunction, commonly called ED in polite society. That means they can't get it up.

ED is three times more common in diabetic men than in non-diabetic men, it hits at a much younger age, and of course it becomes more prevalent and severe the older you get. I won't scare you with the exact statistical details and odds against you in the long run.

Several things you need to know: ED medications *may* work, but are significantly less likely to work than in non-diabetic men. So the little blue pill may or may not save you.

Are all the clouds on your erotic horizon dark? No. The best thing you can do to keep your penis up is to keep your blood sugar down. Keeping your blood pressure in normal range is good too, both for erectile function and for not having a heart attack in a sleazy hotel with a cheap streetwalker. That type of thing always makes your wife look bad and makes your conservative constituents angry.

Now excuse me ladies, I need to talk to all the guys over here in the corner for a minute. Guys, if it is already too late for you, or if you lose to the steep odds, I have a couple of tips for you. *Don't be selfish bastards.* Without crossing the line into becoming a sex manual for diabetics (….although….maybe my next book….), there is more than one way to satisfy a woman. Do not shut the door on intimacy if you develop ED. Talk to your partner. Work something out. *In sickness and in health* is a vow for married folks and a good guiding principle for other relationships. You are in this together, right?

OK, ladies, you can come back into the room now. So speaking of the cost of diabetes in the bedroom, let's touch on the cost of diabetes in the bank account.

Dollars and sense

Endocrinologist JoEllen Habas, MD, said it best: "Diabetes is a pain. A pain in the neck. A pain in the finger tips. And a pain the wallet."

So test strips, blood sugar meds, all of these other meds, doctor's visits, lab tests…what the *fuck* is this all going to cost me? For God's sake don't add it up. It will depress you.

But seeing as how you've taken your anti-depressant today, I'll tell you that our friends over at the ADA actually do keep track of this kind of stuff. Their latest estimate is $11,744 per year. It will be more if you are a T-1.

Of course, no one really pays that much. If you have insurance, diabetes will still hit you in the wallet, but your insurance company will pay for at least *part* of everything. If you don't have insurance you will almost certainly be forced to cut corners on your health care which *will* cut years off of your life. But you may simply have no choice. Because of my somewhat high profile in the online T-1 community, I get emails every day on this subject that would make you break down and cry.

Alcohol and diabetes

At this sobering point, we could all use a drink. I personally don't have a drinking problem. I drink. I get drunk. I fall down. No problem.

OK, that was just a joke. I do have three vices, and heavy drinking is not one of them. *For those of you dying of curiosity, my vices are (1) I drink expensive coffee, (2) I smoke a pipe, (3) and I'm sure this one will come as a huge surprise to you—I swear*. I gave up wild women and song a while back; and I take too many prescription drugs to think recreational drugs would be any fun at all. Gambling has no appeal for me; being diabetic is risk enough.

So you drink. It can be beer, wine, or the good….er….hard… stuff. All have varying degrees of alcohol. Once the alcohol hits your stomach it goes into the bloodstream. Then where does it go? You've probably never thought about it, but I bet you can figure it out. What organ gets wiped out first in alcoholics? Yep, the multi-tasking liver takes the fall.

The liver is the alcohol filter in your body. And now for something you probably didn't know: it is also the insulin filter. Yep, the liver filters out unused, unneeded insulin. Unless it is busy filtering out alcohol. Apparently, when the liver is drunk it doesn't multi-task so well.

Even non-diabetic people will see their blood sugar drop after drinking. If you've got basal insulin pulsing through your circulatory system, drinking alcohol will have the effect of increasing the insulin's potency. I call it the *Jack Daniels Bolus*.

You can, in fact, lower hyperglycemia with alcohol. I don't recommend it, however, as the results can be…unpredictable. Damn. There goes the book *Controlling Your Diabetes with Jack*, the CD's, the workshops… Oh well.

I do love a glass of red wine (or two) with dinner now and again. Probably more now than again. *I think I mentioned that I'm a poor role model.* There is some evidence that red wine is good for the heart, so it's really medicine, right? I don't care for beer myself, but again, a beer with dinner isn't going to hurt you, nor will a margarita.

However, if you drink a lot of beer, like my "light" drinker who puts down 14 beers in a night, the pickling of your liver will only be one of your problems. An average 12-ounce can of beer has 150 calories (beers actually vary from a low of 95 to a high of 209 depending on brand and type). If you drink 14 beers that's 2,100 calories; one-hundred more calories than the recommended *total* daily calories for an adult. Even if you don't eat any food *ever*, with this extra 100 calories per day you will still gain ten pounds in a year by drinking that much beer.

Bottom line: beer can make you fat. If you are fat your insulin resistance increases. If your insulin resistance increases.....

If you drink in moderation, especially with food, and are aware that the drink could cause your blood sugar to drop—especially a few hours downstream—then by all means enjoy all that life has to offer.

Drugs, not the kind you get a prescription for

Which brings us to recreational drugs. *Are you out of your fucking mind?!* Don't you have enough trouble without likely damage to your body, the expense, and the possibility of finding yourself in jail?! If you must smoke pot, snort cocaine, eat funky mushrooms, do meth, or shoot heroin with your insulin syringes, at least do so in moderation and recruit a designated blood sugar checker who is *not* stoned. If you are high, low, or passed out you will not check your blood sugar. You will not be at your mental best either, to say the least. You, can, in fact, die. Beyond the fact you'll be too out of it to test, or probably even understand the numbers (wow....man....a 32...cool...); the drugs themselves can, **and do** have unpredictable effects on your blood sugar. I don't make a habit of preaching abstinence from anything….but aren't you already taking enough drugs?

Diabetes and stress

Remember what happens when the moon is in Scorpio, the wind is from the south and the barometric pressure is stable? Right. Your blood sugar does the funky chicken dance.

This, for some D-folk, causes stress. And what does stress do to your blood sugar? Right. So I want to introduce you to one of my guiding principles for surviving and thriving with diabetes: celebrate defeat.

Diabetes control is an art, not a science. No matter how hard you try, sometimes things will still go wrong.

Laugh, don't cry.

Look to see if you can divine why it happened. If you can't, shrug it off. Chalk it up to human nature and the fact that God has a wicked sense of humor; then keep right on trying.

Or maybe you need a vacation.

Taking a vacation from your diabetes

So let's talk about the subject of diabetes vacations. And I don't mean a cruise with D-friendly food, although I think that is a hell of a good idea and I'll be happy to volunteer as a speaker for free so long as you pick up the tab for me, the wife, and the kid.

I'm also not talking about Diabetes Camp, which is a wonderful opportunity for T-1 kiddos where they can do all the camp stuff with their own kind and see that they aren't the only ones that deal with all of this; and where parents don't need to freak out 'cause the adult staff are all T-1s too and know how to take care of the kids.

I'm talking about more of a stress break here. Not too long ago one of our patients was planning to go to Italy for two weeks. I offered to come along to carry her luggage, but she had it under control. Damn.

She is very meticulous about checking her blood sugar. She is on oral pills with a good A1C. Her risk of a hypo is pretty much nil. I told her to leave her meter behind and go have a good time. She cried. From happiness.

She and her husband had a great time. She ate whatever she wanted for two weeks. Yeah, probably her blood sugar went up a little, but she didn't know, or care, and she had two weeks of "normal" life again.

She still took her meds, but she left her diabetes back home in the drawer of her nightstand with her meter. I think, within the limits of personal safety, that diabetes vacations are a great idea and I think you should get out your day planner, PDA, or smart phone right now and schedule one.

Our computer guy at the clinic is not D-folk. Not yet. He's Hispanic (read higher risk), overweight (read higher-higher risk), but young (read lower risk). That said, he decided the time had come to lose some weight. He's taking his diet very seriously, but he gives himself one day per week "off" to eat whatever the hell he wants. It keeps him focused on the other six days, and it keeps him from falling off the wagon altogether.

It works for him, and we're all proud of him. For D-folks a weekly vacation is probably a bit too much for good long-term health, but taking one day per month or one day every six weeks to feed your *Id* is a good idea. If you are somewhat careful, the worst that can happen is that your blood sugar will go up, you'll be a grump, and feel like crap the next day; but in two or three days you'll be back to your normal control-machine self. You will have done no lasting harm and there is a lot to be said for occasionally feeding the soul, even at the expense of the body. It makes life full and worthwhile.

Smoking

Speaking of worthwhile, I just love relaxing at the end of the day on my porch smoking a pipe. No smoking is healthy, let's be clear about that. At least smoking a pipe is a bit less worse than smoking cigarettes because the smoke is "puffed." The smoke stays in your mouth, and never gets down into your lungs. But I couldn't really advocate it. But both to avoid being a hypocrite, and as part of my one-step-at-a-time philosophy, I'm not too hard on cigarette smokers.

The newly diagnosed, and highly depressed patient looks at me sadly: "Does this mean I'll have to stop smoking too?"

Me: Let's just take this one step at a time. There are a lot of health benefits to quitting smoking; but a lot is changing in your life right now and I don't want to add to your stress, which will just make your blood sugar worse. Why don't you just cut back one or two cigarettes per day for now and we'll worry about it later? If and when you want to quit totally I've got some programs that can help.

Having said all of that, I'm going to give you some FACTS from the Surgeon General and the American Cancer Society about what happens inside your body when you quit smoking cigarettes, bearing in mind that I'm a pipe-smoking hypocrite who recently told my wife to bury me with at least one of my pipes:

- 20 minutes after your last cigarette your blood pressure drops to normal, your pulse rate falls to normal levels, and your body temperature in your hands and feet rises to normal.

- 8 hours after your last cigarette the carbon dioxide level in your blood drops to normal and the oxygen level in your blood returns to normal levels.

- 24 hours after your last cigarette your chance of a heart attack drops measurably.

- 48 hours after your last cigarette nerve endings start to re-grow, increasing your ability to smell and taste.

- 72 hours after your last cigarette your body is free of nicotine, your bronchial tubes relax and your lung capacity increases.

- 2 weeks after your last cigarette your circulation improves, walking becomes easier again.

- 3 months after your last cigarette your lung function has increased by 30%.

- Within 9 months coughing, sinus congestion, fatigue and shortness of breath decrease. You have more energy.

- 1 year after your last cigarette your risk of coronary heart disease is half that of a smoker.

- 5 years after your last cigarette your risk of stroke is the same as a nonsmoker.

- 10 years after your last cigarette your lung cancer risk is now half that of a smoker.

- 15 years after your last cigarette your risk of heart disease in now back to that of a nonsmoker.

Anyway. It is up to you to decide how much pleasure you get out of smoking vs. how many fewer years you want be on the planet to pay for that pleasure.

You know, that statement came out a bit more manipulative than I had intended, because I meant it sincerely. Why live forever if you are frickin' miserable? I guess my big objection to cigarettes is that they not only shorten your life, but reduce the quality of that life while they kill you. Full disclosure: I've been a cigarette smoker at various times of my life.

I guess, as it came up in that list of what cigarettes do *to* you (logically correlating the inverse from the data of what quitting does *for* you), it makes sense to touch on hypertension once again.

High blood pressure and other things that cause trouble

Little-known but important fact: all D-folk worry about what diabetes will do to their kidneys. It is true that high blood sugar will devastate your kidneys. In time. But what many people don't realize is that hypertension will do it even more quickly, and if you have both high blood sugar and high blood pressure…well, you better just call your local dialysis center right now and reserve a bed. You are going to need it.

There is a wonderful word my boss likes to use: *co-morbidities*. He actually used it once during my initial job interview. I had never heard it before and freaked out under my skin. Of course I just nodded and smiled and prayed I could bluff my way through the interview without his realizing what a complete idiot I really am. As soon as I got home I Googled it.

Co-morbidities are other medical conditions that exist in connection with, or in conjunction with the primary illness. Remember that diabetes doesn't like to play alone? There is more than one horseman in the apocalypse!

Diabetes co-morbidities include: all of the "pathies" (neuropathy, retinopathy, nephropathy, bummeropathy), hypertension, hyperlipidima, depression. We've got enough horsemen to make up a Cavalry regiment!

To live a full, happy, and healthy life as a diabetic, you need to control more than your diabetes. You need to keep all the horsemen in check.

Speaking of horseback riding, which always conjures up a 1950s scene of a family at a dude ranch in Arizona for me…no idea why, we never did that…I want to talk to you about your family. They are your largest asset *for*, and your largest challenge *to* controlling your diabetes.

La Familia

I hooked up with one of our state's top endos (not in *that* way), who practiced at a major medical center in Albuquerque, the closest thing we have to a metropolis. My goal was to "shadow" her like some sort of knowledge-sucking vampire. A couple of times a month I made the four-hour round-trip drive to the city—leaving in the dark before sunup and coming home again in the moonlight. I put a lot of gas in my Honda and a lot of Starbucks in my blood.

One day we had a poorly-controlled young female T-1 come in. I didn't detect anything unusual about the visit, but after my kinswoman had left, the doctor shook her head. "Well, that patient is a lost cause," she sighed.

Huh? Why?

"Because she came to the appointment by herself. She either has no family to support her, or they don't care enough to be actively engaged in her diabetes."

Wow. Ever since then, I get a rush when the T-3s come with their loved ones to my office for appointments. And damned if the ones who come with family don't do better.

Oh, gosh, so where to even begin on the delicate subject of family? There is no larger environmental influence on a diabetic than his or her family. They can support, tempt, help or hinder your health. This is why the concept of Type-3 diabetics is *sooooooo* important: you do not have diabetes all by yourself; your entire family has it too. Whether they like it or not.

And some do *not* like it. Way too many diabetics, at best, have to watch their loved ones continue to suck down regular soda, eat high-carb meals, and wallow in candy bars. At worst they might live with families who push them to join; "Come on, one Coke won't kill you."

The good thing about eating healthy for diabetes is that it is the same as eating healthy for anyone. Healthy eating is healthy eating. It is the same for diabetics and for non-diabetics. If your family joins you in eating healthy for your diabetes, they will actually be eating healthy for themselves too. Everyone wins.

The next worst fate, after a family that doesn't give a shit, is one that cares *too* much, but doesn't have the facts.

"Can you eat that?"

"You shouldn't eat that!"

"I read in the National Enquirer that if you take crushed stingray tail you can cure your diabetes."

"Your grandmother (grandfather, aunt, great uncle, father) had diabetes and went blind after starting insulin, that stuff will kill you!"

Some families have had intergenerational negative experiences with diabetes. To them, the end game is unavoidable. Diabetes is a death sentence and it doesn't matter what you do so you might as well eat cheesecake.

Realistically, there is not a hell of a lot you can do about your family. Hopefully you have a strong, loving, supportive one. If not, your best option is to at least *try* to educate them. Teach them about what you need to do and why. *Ask* them to help you, and to support you.

Twinkies and corn chips, a world of temptation

The last topic I want to cover in the real world is Lucifer's Amusement Park: Carb-Land. One of my bosses (I have a couple) has a carb addiction. One of her self-enablement strategies is to bring treats for her crew. By doing this, she isn't really buying the chocolate-lemon-fudge bunt cake for *herself*, she's buying it for *her whole crew*. The diabetes ed building is an old modular at the end of the clinic's parking lot. I spend a lot of time every day going back and forth from my building to the main clinic. It's great exercise for me and so long as it isn't snowing, raining, or freezing cold with hurricane-strength winds, I don't mind.

But as I come into the clinic's back door, I go past her office. Across the hall from her office is the table I've nicknamed *the carb table*. And what do we have today? Ah, M&Ms. Yesterday it was homemade chocolate chip cookies. Tomorrow it will be, God help me, Entenmann's doughnuts.

Once, after eating *three* Rich Chocolate Entenmann's doughnuts at a staff meeting, I compared myself to a disgraced televangelist: I know the Word; I preach the Word; I even believe the Word. But still, I'm in the back room screwing the church secretary.

I think I mentioned that I'm a poor role model.

No single thing in my life has been worse for my diabetes than getting a job working in the health care industry. Ironic. A little at a time I have small victories. At Halloween we now give out healthy snacks…well, healthier, anyway. Staff meetings feature more fruit than pastries. But still, all of us, D-folk and normal mortals alike, love sweets.

About a week ago I was able to walk past not one, but two different kinds of brownies for most of the day. Then, probably from the chocolate aroma molecules floating in the chaos-laden air, in the mid-afternoon my blood sugar mysteriously spiked to 225. Well, I'm high anyway…give me a frickin' brownie!

Oh, and by the way, the ones with powdered sugar were better than the ones without—I had to try both for purely scientific purposes.

If you watch TV in the evenings, you will be bombarded by pictures of food. Pizza, waffles, burgers, pizza again, the never-ending Pasta Bowl at Olive Garden, breakfast cereal, and pizza a third time.

It would be a lot easier to eat healthy on a deserted island than it is on the carb-soaked streets of America. My advice…. Well, crap. Maybe I don't have any. How good is your willpower?

I guess it boils down to try your best and don't beat yourself up if and when you fail. And if you fail, it doesn't mean you have to stay in a state of failure. Pick yourself up and start over again!

Some doctors, many diabetes educators, and most nutritionists tend to forget that there is something out there called *the real world*. If you live in a bubble on top of a mountain all by yourself you can be perfectly healthy. But the rest of us are in the Garden of Eden with waaaaaay too many snakes and apple trees.

There is a tradition in diabetes health care of blaming the patient for failure. If your doctor tells you to do this-that-and-the-other-thing to lower your blood sugar and you fail, you are branded a "non-compliant" diabetic. Our diagnosis codes for diabetes even classify you as *in* or *out* of control. Somehow I think the video *Diabetics Gone Wild* won't sell quite as well as the *Girls Gone Wild* series.

So my bottom line is this: life is too short for guilt. Recognize the fact that you are a social creature who lives in a less-than-diabetes-friendly environment. While it is true that you are in control, that you are in the driver's seat, there are also forces at play that are greater than you are. Do the best you can, most of the time, and don't let the bastards get you down.

"Gary, you are gonna finish your dessert, and you are gonna like it!"

SpongeBob Squarepants
Cartoon Character

Section 6—Ready, Set, Go!

Chapter 14—Time to cross the finish line .... Page 183

You and I will wrap everything up with the importance of not going it alone. You need support, and what better kind than from your own kind? I'll tell you where and how to find a support group. We'll also cover what to do when you fail and we'll take a look back at everything we've covered on our journey together.

    Support groups—you are not alone .... Page 184
    Getting back on the "wagon" .... Page 184
    It's a wrap! .... Page 185

> "One night after I ate my dinner I was munching on cereal, and as I was stuffing my mouth full of unbolused for carbohydrates, I wondered just how many grams could it possibly be? So I checked... For each "handful" of cheerios I was inhaling, I was eating about 8 grams of carbohydrates. Stunned, I sat there and thought about how many handfuls I would mindlessly eat in one sitting. Four? Five? Eight? Holy crap batman!"

Scott Johnson, Type-1 Diabetic
Computer Guru & Blogger

Chapter 14—Time to cross the finish line

My office is like the air traffic control tower at Kennedy. I'm booked solid from the second I walk in and water my plant until the sun sets and I shut off the lights and lock the door. The phone rings at least six times per hour and I always interrupt what I'm doing to answer it—because once the T-3 of a patient having a life-threatening hypo left a message for me to please call back as soon as I could. She didn't call 911 for an ambulance, but sat by the phone waiting for my call back.

There are walk-ins. Emergencies. Newly dx'd patients. It's absolute chaos. *God, I love it.*

Riiiiiiing! I pause mid-sentence, glancing at the caller ID as I pick up the receiver. It is Nurse's Station 4 calling. I hold up one finger to my patient in the universal sign language of "wait one second." My patients have adjusted to the chaos of their visits and it doesn't even seem unusual to them anymore. *Annex*, I say, knowing that the call is internal. It's the medical director's nurse. "Is this the diabetes cheerleader?" she asks me with a laugh in her voice.

I'm sooooo putting that on my business cards next time.

Support groups—you are not alone

It is good to be a diabetes cheerleader. It is also good to have one at your side, cheering you on. That's why bar-none, one of the best things you can do for yourself (beyond checking your blood sugar, taking all your meds, and eating sensibly) is to join a support group. If you are a T-2, I can pretty much guarantee you'll have one in your community. If you are T-1 you may have to resort to an online support group; but don't discount how powerful these can be. Some of my most favorite people in the world, some of those dearest to my heart, are cyber friends I've never met in the flesh. We share a bond of common experience, and it turns out that the internet can be a surprisingly intimate place.

Support groups can give you a chance to unload your baggage, to see that you are not the only one with the problems you have, facing the challenges you face. You also get to help others, and in doing so you help yourself. They keep you informed, updated, educated, and most importantly they show you that far from being alone, you are part of a tribe.

Getting back on the "wagon"

I also want you to know that no matter how far you've slipped, no matter how damaged your body, you can make it better. If your legs have been cut off and you are blind and on dialysis, you can still turn things around and improve your lot in life. In diabetes, you can always make it better. I promise you.

It's a wrap!

My charter at the beginning of this book was to ***remind you of the things you forgot, update you on the things that have changed, and teach you the things you never learned.*** Let me look back and make sure I've accomplished everything I set out to do.

We covered the various types of diabetics that make up our growing tribe, and we scared ourselves by looking closely at the various risks associated with poor control: the innocuous-sounding *complications*. We talked about your best personal tool in this battle: home glucose monitoring. Together we discussed how to use the machines, when to test and what the numbers mean. We reviewed high and low blood sugars and the warnings and dangers associated with them. We even peeked into the future to see what it will be like when you know what your blood sugar is doing all the time!

We deciphered the A1C test and showed how stable, low blood sugars head off complications at the pass. We delved into the relationship between food and your blood sugar and then went on to look at how every frickin' thing in the world affects your blood sugar too. We covered the importance of weight loss for those people whose spouses keep shrinking their laundry. (My pants are too tight, the damn woman must'a shrunk them in the laundry! What? Oh, three corn dogs for me, Hon.) And how to lose that weight.

We talked about why your blood pressure and lipids matter, and how important your heart's health is as a diabetic. We reviewed the medications for blood sugar in perhaps painful detail with all those multi-syllabic words that look both unpronounceable and un-understandable—and on top of that we covered the other meds you need to *ask your doctor* about.

For those of you injecting, we reviewed injection technique; which also served as a primer for those of you who don't inject yet, and I hope I convinced you that it is really no big fucking deal at all. And last we talked about the challenges of the real world in which all of us D-folk and our families live.

I think it has been a nice little journey, and I hope you learned a lot without even realizing you were learning. That was my goal, you know. I love to teach, but I personally have a low tolerance for boredom. I wanted you to have fun, enjoy the read, and then say: "Wait a cotton pickin' minute! He tricked me! I learned a bunch of stuff!" If I did that, I earned my title as a Diabetes Educator.

I'm sure as soon as this book goes to print I'll think of 12 things I forgot to talk about, but that's the nature of knowledge. My boss, once sharing a new medical tidbit with me said, his eyes twinkling with delight, "That's why we call it the *practice* of medicine." He wakes full of energy every day in the knowledge he'll learn something new by day's end. I don't wake up full of energy (not my style) but I'll often tell patients: *If you don't learn something new today you might as well have stayed in bed.*

But his lesson to me that day has stuck in my head: medicine is too broad in its scope to be *mastered*; it must be *practiced*.

Likewise, diabetes—divinely complex, always dynamic on its own, always revealing a little more of its dark character to science every day—must be practiced. You may never master diabetes, but if you practice good control you will live a long, healthy, and happy life.

> "Managing your diabetes enables you to fufill all your other obligations and enjoy all that life has to offer."

Gary Scheiner, MS, CDE, Type-1 Diabetic
Diabetes Educator & Author

Final thoughts...

I had another life once, before diabetes. Having diabetes is like living in Dog Years. Time warps, days seem like weeks. Weeks seem like months. Months seem like years and years seem like decades. It is the unrelenting 24-7-365 nature of the disease. I can hardly remember my life as a businessman anymore. It is lost to me in the fog of time past.

For a long time I metaphorically banged my head on the wall: why on earth did this happen to me? Why did diabetes so unexpectedly come to me out of the blue? I'm not really a very religious man, but I am spiritual and after my years at my clinic—after day after day, after day of being able to help "my kind" to be healthier and happier, I've come to believe that this was my destiny. The hand of fate, or God, or providence or whatever you want to call it.

My big sister connected me with a quote from Frederick Buechner that I liked so much I printed it in fancy font on colored paper and hung it on the wall next to my desk. It reads: "The place God calls you to is the place where your deep joy and the world's deep hunger meet." Amen brother.

I was raised a WASP but fell in love with and married a wonderful Hispanic Catholic woman. I wasn't sure how she felt about my going into the medical world until she bought me a *Santo*, a flat piece of wood with the image of a saint on it. In this case, St. Agatha, patron of nurses. It was her way of saying: *go for it*.

The day of my first clinical I was up before dawn, scared to death. I got into my scrubs and put my stethoscope around my neck. The great thing about a stethoscope is that you look like you know what you are doing even when you are scared and ignorant. I took the Santo off of the wall and fingered it gently.

I didn't want to screw up. I wanted to be compassionate, smart, and capable. From nowhere a little prayer popped into my head, and to this day I start and end each day with it. I wanted to share it here with you, at the end of this book.

So here's my little prayer as a diabetes educator—

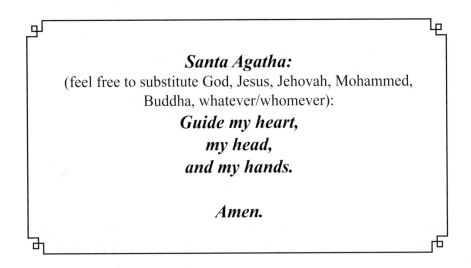

Santa Agatha:
(feel free to substitute God, Jesus, Jehovah, Mohammed, Buddha, whatever/whomever):
*Guide my heart,
my head,
and my hands.*

Amen.

Acknowledgements

It is tradition bordering on unwritten *law* that acknowledgements are placed at the beginning of a book. As always, I've chosen to do things a little differently. I have placed them at the back—not out of disrespect, quite the contrary.

Once you read this book, those who influence me and help me will be of greater interest to you than they would have been when you first opened the book.

Now, I have to tell you that it scares the shit out of me even to attempt to compile a list of all the people that helped shape this book in one form or another; I live in terror that I'll forget someone to whom I owe a debt of gratitude. Sometimes the most obvious things slip past, like the typo in our subtitle that went unnoticed until nearly the final draft. So, to make sure I don't miss the most obvious, I'll start with….my mother.

Thanks, **Mom,** for your huge help with editing the first draft…. and the second… and the third… and the…

To my dear friend, colleague, and mentor of sorts—and author of this book's forward—**Dr. Colleran**.

To **Dr. Young** for having such faith in me and giving me so many opportunities; and to **Sig** for giving me a job where I can contribute… and for not firing me from the same on a number of occasions.

To **"Dr." Elaine** and **Dr. Ruiz**; my dear friends, colleagues, and carpooling buddies to distant training opportunities.

To all my **Co-workers** and **Colleagues** at the clinic; surely the brightest and most dedicated medical team ever assembled anywhere.

To **Dr. Habas, Dr. Grant, Dr. Pinon, Dr. Olivares.**

To my gang of *Diabetes Peer Educators* who work so hard for me: **Angelina, Alice, Charlotte, Jim, Richard, Rick,** and **Tahirih.**

To the health blogosphere and especially my e-friends **Amy, Six,** and **Scott.**

To "my" **Patients**, who teach me so very much by letting me teach them.

To **Jane** and **Jane**, both the one who was instrumental in connecting me to my current job, and the one who is my right-hand woman who keeps my operation running smoothly.

To **Rajivi** and all the other assorted geniuses and experts out there who contribute to the knowledge of diabetes every day.

And of course, to my wife, Debbie.

Resources

On the web:
I start every day with Starbucks Coffee. After that I go to:

http://www.diabetesmine.com
This is the "blog" of Amy Tenderich. I put *blog* in quotes because her website is sooooo much more than a blog. Amy is a professional journalist who was dx'd with T-1 as an adult. Her site is the *New York Times* of diabetes. If you want to know what's going on in the research, politics, and economics of diabetes this is where you need to be.

http://www.sixuntilme.com
This is the blog of Kerri Morrone Sparling, one of my best e-friends. She's just a joy to read. You won't feel like the only one with diabetes if you spend your morning with her.

http://www.diabetestalkfest.ning.com
Try this site for online support and sense of community.

http://www.lifeafterdx.blogspot.com
This is the author's blog. I'm pretty sloppy about posting nowadays, but if you want to learn about Continuous Glucose Monitoring scroll back to the beginning. This is the *War and Peace* of CGM. I documented every day of my time as a CGM pioneer for months. More recent posts deal with my various favorite soapbox issues.

http://www.redbloodcellbooks.com
This is the home page of this book's publisher! It's a fun and funky (no, really) website. It is also the best place to keep an eye out for my next book.

In print:
There are dozens of magazines and hundreds of books about diabetes. My favorite magazine is:

Diabetes Health, P.O. Box 395, Woodacre, CA 94973 (800) 234-1218 online at *www.diabeteshealth.com*.

In the trenches:
Our two biggest organizations are:

The **American Diabetes Association** (ADA), fighting the good fight mainly at the legislative and research levels. I'm glad we have them, but their only interest in *you* is as a source of funds. Find them at *www.diabetes.org* or (800) 342-2383.

The **Juvenile Diabetes Research Foundation** (JDRF), searching and funding cure research for T-1. Find them at *www.jdfr.org* or (800) 533-2873.

Glossary

ACE—a.k.a. **ACE Inhibitor**. Angiotensin-Converting Enzyme, a high blood pressure pill that can help protect your kidneys from high blood sugar.

ADA—the American Diabetes Association.

Adrenaline—a flight-or-fight hormone that can cause blood sugar to rise. Its function is to give you a short burst of extra energy in life-threatening situations, but modern day stress can cause a steady "drip" of adrenaline that can make blood sugar control tricky.

AGI—Alpha-glucosidase Inhibitors. A Class of oral diabetes drugs that block the absorption of carbohydrates in the small intestines.

A1C—a.k.a. **HbA1c** or **A1c**. A blood test used to assess the overall level of blood sugar control.

Autoimmune—failure of the body to recognize its own parts.

Beta cells—the pancreatic cells that produce the hormone insulin.

BGL—Blood Glucose Level, also sometimes called your blood sugar level, or simply blood sugar.

BMI—Body Mass Index. A ratio of height to weight that gives a rough framework for judging if a person is overweight, correct weight for height, or underweight.

Bolus—a shot of insulin, usually to cover a meal, but also used with corrections: correction bolus.

Capillary—the smallest blood vessels, found in fingers, toes, eyes, and kidneys.

Carbohydrates—a simple sugar. High carb foods impact blood sugar quickly. Examples include all sugars, flour, pasta, and starches.

Carbs—slang for carbohydrates.

CGM—Continuous Glucose Monitoring. A system that checks your blood sugar hundreds of times per day.

Chronic—permanent.

DPP-4—an enzyme in the incretin family whose job it is to stop the action of GLP-1.

DKA—Diabetic Ketoacidosis. A life threatening coma-like condition caused by the buildup of ketones in the blood when blood sugar is high. Most common in T-1 diabetics, but any diabetic can "go" DKA.

dLife—a diabetes media empire that includes a popular TV show and website.

DNA—Deoxyribonucleic acid, the biological genetic blueprint that makes you who you are, with all your strengths and weaknesses.

Dx—a.k.a. **dx'd**. Slang for diagnosed. Often used in reference to the day a diabetic learns he or she *is* diabetic.

ED—Erectile Dysfunction. Impotence caused by a medical condition.

Edema—the swelling of tissues, caused by retention of fluid.

EMT—Emergency Medical Technician. Yeah, the guys in the ambulance.

Endocrinologist—a medical doctor who specializes in treating various conditions of the endocrine system, diabetes amongst them.

Epidermis—your skin.

Excursion—a rapid change in blood sugar levels, especially upwards.

FDA—Food and Drug Administration. The folks who, among many other things, approve new drugs for the U.S. market.

Genetic predisposition—meaning that the basic blueprint of your genetic code makes you more likely to have certain conditions, traits, or diseases.

GLP-1—an incretin that controls the speed of digestion and contributes to the sensation of satiety—feeling full when you eat.

Glucometer—a.k.a. **Glucose Meter**. A small device used to measure the level of sugar in your blood.

Glucose—a simple sugar that is the basic fuel for the human body. The digestive system converts everything you eat to glucose.

Glucagon Emergency Kit—a hormone shot designed to revive a person who has lost consciousness from low blood sugar.

HDL—the "good" cholesterol.

Hormone—a chemical messenger. Various parts of the body use hormones to communicate with each other. Think of it as your cell phone plan for your cells.

Hyperglycemia—a.k.a. **Hyper**. High blood sugar. Usually defined as above 200 mg/dl.

Hyperlipidmia—high lipids (such as cholesterol and triglycerides).

Hypertension—high blood pressure.

Hypoglycemia—a.k.a. **Hypo**. Low blood sugar. Usually defined as below 75 mg/dl.

Id—Sigmund Freud's psychotherapy classification of the impulsive, childlike portion of the psyche that operates on the "pleasure principle," notorious for doing only what it wants with no regard for consequences.

Immune system—the body's defense system against infection.

Incretin(s)—a newly understood class of complex hormones and enzymes that play a major role in digestion.

Injectables—drugs that must be taken by injection. A shot.

Insulin—a hormone that allows the body to move glucose out of the bloodstream and into cells.

Insulin Resistance—a condition in which the body's cells don't respond normally to insulin.

Interstitial fluid—the "water" between cells.

Ketone—a by-product of cells burning fat when they can't get glucose. When ketones build up in the blood they change the pH, causing the blood to become more acid.

LDL—"bad" cholesterol.

LFT—Liver Function Test, a blood test to evaluate the overall health of the liver.

Lipids—a broad category of various blood fats and cholesterol.

Metabolize—a body process for converting food to fuel, often carbs to energy.

Microalbumin—small protein molecules. Their presence in urine is the first warning sign of kidney failure.

Molecule—the smallest particle of a substance that retains the character of the substance. If you get any smaller, it's just parts.

Monotherapy—using only one drug or therapy to address a health issue.

Nephropathy—kidney complications.

Neuropathy—nerve damage complications.

Orals—slang for pills. Medications taken by mouth.

Pancreas—an organ located just behind your stomach that produces insulin.

Pineal Gland—an endocrine gland deep inside the brain that may regulate sleep patterns.

Postprandial—medical-speak for "after eating."

Predisposed—meaning you are more likely to develop a condition, usually genetically.

Progressive—continuing to get worse over time.

PWD—Person With Diabetes.

Rebound excursion—a high blood sugar caused by over-correcting a low blood sugar.

Renal failure—a.k.a. End Stage Renal Disease or ESRD. Failure of the kidneys. Dialysis is required for survival.

Retinopathy—eye complications which can lead to blindness.

Serotonin—a hormone that is connected to depression.

Statins— a class of cholesterol-lowering drugs.

Thyroid—a gland in the throat that controls the body's metabolic rate.

Titration—slowly and steadily changing a medication to let the body adjust until the therapeutic goal is reached.

TSH—a blood test to check thyroid function.

WTF?—blog slang for What The Fuck?

"What you put in your mouth can only help or hurt YOU—not your health care provider, and certainly not your diabetes educator.

I tell this to my patients all the time. Think about what is going into your mouth before putting it in."

Elaine Montaño, MSN, CNP, Type-1
Health Care Provider

Bibliography

This really isn't a traditional kind of *biblio* because I'm really not a traditional kind of author and this isn't really a traditional kind of book. As an educator I read books, magazines, and studies constantly, attend every seminar I can, scour the internet, and basically just absorb all the information I come across like some sort of psychotic sponge—but I don't really do a very good job of keeping track of where I get information from. I'm more of a clinical storm trooper than an academician. And much medical information appears in so many respected sources that it would take a detective the likes of Sherlock Holmes to discover the source of origin.

I've asked two medical professionals for whom I have the absolute highest respect to read this book for medical accuracy. I am quite confident that all the medical "facts" are current and accurate by today's medical standards. Every day diabetes reveals more of its dark face to us, and every day our scientists probe deeper into the timeless mysteries of human biology and physiology.

My readers are:

Kathleen Colleran, MD, *Endocrinologist, Associate Professor of Medicine, University of New Mexico HSC, Albuquerque, New Mexico.*

Dr. C, being both a clinician and a researcher, is not so sure that diabetes is actually progressive. She believes that under perfect, controlled conditions, diabetes would stay stable. That said, I see diabetes progress daily in the real world and even she will concede that diabetes is "functionally" progressive if not biologically so.

***Elaine Montaño, MSN, CNP**, Certified in Advanced Diabetes Care, Medical Director and Owner of LifeCare Health Services, LLC, Santa Fe, New Mexico, and a T-1 herself.*

Elaine is quick to point out when statements like "most diabetics die of heart attacks" are thrown around, that it is *out-of-control diabetics* that die of heart attacks. While that is true, it is also still true that statistically heart attacks do kill most diabetics, which in turn tells us that most diabetics are not in control.

Faced with the problem of giving credit where credit is due, I decided to list in the Bibliography the contents of my library. These are the books that have had the greatest impact on my knowledge base and thinking processes. If I left out someone, I apologize. It is not my goal to steal, only to teach.

The books are:

Bernstein, Richard K. *Dr. Bernstein's Diabetes Solution. The complete guide to achieving normal blood sugars.* New York, Little, Brown and Company, 2007

Diabetes Care. American Diabetes Association: Clinical Practice Recommendations 2008. USA, American Diabetes Association, 2008

Edelman, Steven V., et al. *Diagnosis and Management of Type 2 Diabetes*. New York, Professional Communications, Inc. 2008

Edelman, Steven V., et al. *Taking Control of Your Diabetes, Third Edition*. New York, Professional Communications, Inc. 2007

Hazlett, James. *The Best of Diabetes Self-Management, the definitive commonsense guide to managing your diabetes*. New York, Diabetes Self-Management Books, 2002

Hirsch, James S. *Cheating Destiny: Living with Diabetes, America's Biggest Epidemic*. Houghton Mifflin Company, 2006

Jackson, Richard and Tenderich, Amy. *Know Your Numbers, Outlive your Diabetes: 5 essential health factors you can master to enjoy a long and healthy life*. New York, The Marlowe Diabetes Library, 2007

Kaufman, Francine R. *Diabesity: What you need to know if anyone you care about suffers from weight problems, pre-diabetes, or diabetes*. New York, Bantam Books, 2006

Marieb, Elaine N. *Human Anatomy & Physiology, Sixth Edition*. San Francisco, Pearson Benjamin Cummings, 2004

National Diabetes Information Clearinghouse. *The Diabetes Dictionary*. NIH Publication No. 02-3016, 2002

New Mexico Health Care Takes on Diabetes. *New Mexico Diabetes Practice Guideline*. New Mexico, NMTOD, 2008

NIH and CDC. *Diabetes: The Numbers*. On-line, 2007

O'Keefe, James H. Jr., et al. *Diabetes Essentials, Second Edition*. Michigan, Physician's Press, 2005

Porth, Carol Mattson. *Pathophysiology: Concepts of altered health states*. Philadelphia, Lippincott Williams & Wilkins, 2002

Rosenbloom, Arlan and Silverstein, Janet H. *Type 2 Diabetes in Children and Adolescents: A guide to diagnosis, epidemiology, pathogenesis, prevention, and treatment*. USA, American Diabetes Association, 2003

Scheiner, Gary. *Think like a pancreas: A practical guide to managing diabetes with insulin*. New York, Marlowe & Company, 2004

Skyler, Jay S., et al. *DiabetesDek, Professional Edition, How to Control and Manage Diabetes Mellitus*. USA, Infodek, 2004, 2007 (14th Ed.)

Tsiaras, Alexander. *The Architecture and Design of Man and Woman*. New York, Doubleday, 2004

Walker, Richard. *Body.* London, DK, 2005

Whalley, Angelina. *Gunther von Hagen's Body Worlds. The anatomical exhibition of real human bodies.* Heidelberg, Germany, 2006

I also used the ADA website at *www.diabetes.org* as a source of data and statistics.

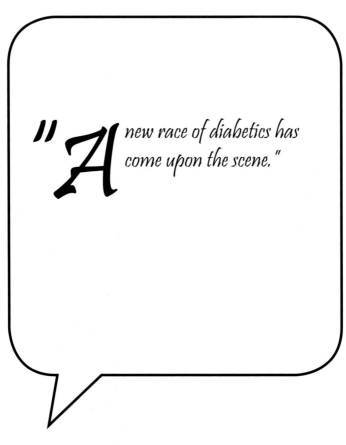

"A new race of diabetics has come upon the scene."

Elliott Joslin, MD
Diabetes Treatment Pioneer, *writing about T-1s shortly after insulin was discovered*

Index

—A—

A1C 61, **65-72**, 185, 109, 185, 195
ACCORD 70
ACE inhibitor **157-159**, 195
AC meals 42
Actos **127**, 128
alcohol 101, 118, 122-123, **165-166**, 146, 166
alcohol pads 37, 39
alert jewelry 5, **46**, 148
Alpha-glucosidase Inhibitors 126
alternate site testing **36-37**, 57
Amaryl 124
AM Fasting 42
amputations 9, **27**, 108
anti-depressants 85
Apidra 140
aspirin 103, **157**
atherosclerosis 100
autoimmune **11**, 14, 195
Avandia 127-130

—B—

baby aspirin 157
Basal/Bolus therapy 141
basal insulin **139-140**, 147, 166
beta cells **11**, 195
BGL *see blood*
blindness **25**, 48, **109**, 176, 184, 201
blood pressure 77, 89, 90, **97-100**, 103, 116, 122, **158-159**, 163, 171, **173-174**, 185
blood **24**, 65
blood sugar 8, 16, **65-66**
  high 16, **23**, 26-27, **47-48**, 85, 86
  low 32, **44-46**, 69, 70, **142**
blood sugar check 31-32, 39-42, **53-54**
  AC meals 42
  AM Fasting 42
  HS 42
  postprandial **42**, 49, 200
  random **42**, 49
blood sugar levels **47**, 56, 58, 67, 71, 85, 86, 138-140, 195

Index

blood sugar targets 55
BMI **95-96**, 196
Body Mass Index **95-96**, 196
bolus **138, 141**, 165, 196
breakfast 42, 49, 63, 66, **107-108**
Byetta 153-155

—C—

caffeine 81
calibrate (meter) **50**, 54
calibration (meter) 50-51
calibration errors (meter) 51
calories 73, 74, **92-94**, 107-108, 138, 167
cannula 150
capillaries **24-25**, 72, 98, **163**
carbohydrates *a.k.a carbs* 61, 71, **74-77**, 85, 121, 126, 131, 138, 140, 141, 149, 151, 176, **177-178**, 195, 196, 200
CGM 29, **55-59**, 193, 196
  calibration 56
  sampling lag 57

cholesterol 77, 89, **101-102**, 103, 106, 159 *also see HDL and LDL*
chronic **8**, 53, 72, 83, 85, 119, 158, 196
cigarette(s) 170-173
combo-therapy 132
co-morbidities 173-174
complications 9, **23-28**, 32, 54, 65, 69, 109, 185, 200, 201
Continuous Glucose Monitors: *see CGM*
continuous monitoring: *see CGM*
Crestor 159

—D—

Davidson, Michael 102
depression 62, **83-85**, 174, 201
Diabesity 92
DiaBeta Micronase 124
Diabetes Control and Complications Trial 69

Index

diabetes, types of:
  Gestational Diabetes 20-21
  Pre-diabetes 19-20
  Type-1 Daibetes 11-14
  Type-1.5 Diabetes 14-15
  Type-2 Diabetes 15-19
  Type-3 Diabetes 21
diabetic ketoacidosis **47**, 196
Diabinese 124
dialysis **26**, 39, 173, 184, 201
diet 18, 61, **73-80**, 91, 94, 100, **118-120**, 121, 130, 138, **158**, 170
dilated eye exam 109
distal capillaries **24-25**, **163**
DKA **47**, 196
dLife **21**, 196
DPP-4 **131**, 153, 196

—E—

eAG 68
ED **163-164**, 197
edema **127-128**, 197
Equal 74

erectile dysfunction **163-164**, 197
estimated average glucose 68
excursions 71-72
exercise 8, 44, 81, **82-83**, **92-94**, 118-120, 121, 130, 177

—F—

family 13, 17, **21**, 73, 78, 161, **175-176**
fast acting insulin 139
fat
  lipid/dietary 45, 47, **77**, 96, **100-101**, 199, 200
  obese **17-18**, 21, **89-91**, 107, 127, 167 *also see obestiy*
FDA 36, 50, 55, 105-106, 130, 155, **197**
fiber 77

—G—

genetics 17
Gestational Diabetes 20-21
Glipizide 124-125
GLP-1 **131**, 153, 198

Index

Glucagon 152-153
glucose **12**, 41, 43, 47, 58, 75, 76, 126, **147**, 152
glucose tabs **45**, 148-149
Glynase 124
Glyset 126

—H—

Habas, JoEllen 164
HbA1c 65, *also see A1C*
HDL cholesterol **100-102**, 198
heart attacks **27**, 70, 77, 85, 93, **97**, 100, 101, 102-103, 128, 129, **157**, 159, 164, 171, **204**
high BGL *see blood sugar*
high blood sugar *see blood sugar*
HS 42
Humalog 140
hyperglycemia (hyper) 47, **198**, *also see blood sugar*
hyperlipidemia 77, **198**
hypertension 77, **100**, 106, **173-174**, 198
hypertensive 98

hypoglycemia (hypos) 44, **198**, *also see blood sugar*

—I—

incretins **130-131**, 153, 155, 199
infection 27, **86-87**, 108, 199
infusion set 150
injectable(s) **115**, 131, **133-155**, 199
injection technique 144-147
insulin 11-12, 14, 16, 44, 47, 115, 124, **136-142**, 199
  basal 139
  bolus 39, 42, **138**
insulin pen 143
insulin pump 150-51
insulin resistance **15-17**, 89, 91, 94, 119, 124-125, **127**, 130, 137-138, 153, 167, 199
interstitial fluid **38**, 55, 57, 199

—J—

Januvia 131-132

Index

—K—

Kaufman, Francine R. 92
ketones **47**, 196, 199

—L—

lactic acidosis 122
LADA 14
lance **36-39**, 52
lancing device **35-36**, 37, 38
Lantus 139
Latent Autoimmune Diabetes in Adults 14
LDL cholesterol 100-103
Leaky Liver Syndrome **41**, 121,
Levemir 139
levothyroxine 104
LFT **127**, 199
lipids 63, 97, **100-103**, 185, 189, 200
Lipitor 159
liver function test **127**, 199
LLS **41**, 121

—M—

MDI **141**, 142, 150-151
medical alert jewelry 5, **46**, 148
Medicare 66
meter 29
  calibration 50
  calibration errors 51
meter number 68
metformin 121, 122, 132
Mevacor 159
microalbumin 26, 158
mis-calibrated meter 51
monotherapy 132
mutiple daily injection **141**, 142, 150-151
multi-vitamin 157, **158**

—N—

nephropathy **26**, 174, 200
neuropathy **27**, 85, 108, 174, 200
nocturnal hepatic glucose release 41
non-compliant **79**, 179
Non-HDL Cholesterol 103

Index

NovoLog 140
NPH 141
NutraSweet 74

—O—

obesity **18-19**, 34, 75
orals 115, **121-132**, 153, 200
osteopenia 90

—P—

pain 27, 36, 81, **83**, 89, 122, 164
pancreas **11**, 16-17, 73, 84, 100, 119, 124-127, 130, 137-138, 151, 155, 200
pancreatitis **100**, 155
pen needle 144
periodontal disease 86
poly-pills 100, **132**
postprandial **42**, 49, 200
Prandin 125
Precose 126
pre-diabetes 9, **19-20**
predisposition 12-13, 17, 197, **201**

progressive **8**, 32, 72, 85, 119, 158, 201
pumps 150-151
PWD 5

—Q—

no index item for this letter

—R—

random (BGL test) **42**, 49
rebound excursion **46**, 69, 70, 201
recreational drugs 165, **167-168**
relative hypoglycemia 45
retinopathy **25**, (**109**), 172, 201

—S—

self-managed diseases 31, **53**, 117
self-titrate 147
serotonin **84**, 201
sex 90, 93-94, 159, **163-164**
smoking 118, 161, **170-173**
soda 45, **73**, 75, 76 149, 159, 176
Splenda 74
Starlix 125

Index

statin 103, 157, **159**, 201
stress 70, 81, 87, 118, **168**, 171, 195
strips *see test strips*
stroke 89, **100**, 157, 172
sugar *see glucose or blood sugar*
sugar-free sodas 74
sulfonylureas 124-126
support groups 184
Symlin 155
symptoms of high blood sugar 16
symptoms of low blood sugar 45
Synthroid 104

—T—

target numbers 55
test strips 33, **34-35**, 40, 42, 48-49, **50-51**, 52, 54, 66, 164
The Rule of 15— 45
thyroid 77, **104-108**, 116, 201
triglycerides 100-101, 198
TSH **104**, 201
Types of diabetes *see diabetes*
TZD **127-130**, 132, 138

—U—

no index item for this letter

—V—

no index item for this letter

—W—

warning signs
  high (blood sugar) 16
  low (blood sugar) 45
weight gain **91**, 128, 138-139
white food rule 75-77

—X—

no index item for this letter

—Y—

yeast infections 87

—Z—

Zocor 159

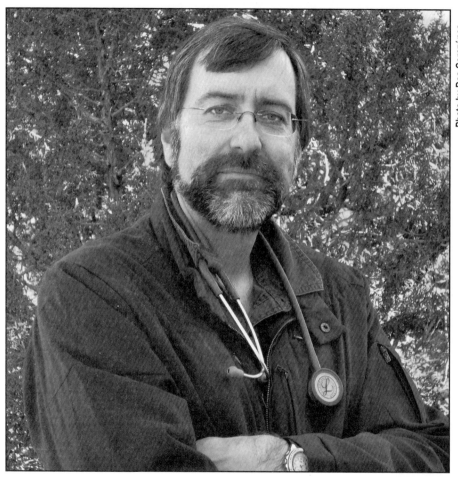

William "Lee" Dubois

About the Author: Type-1 diabetic, diabetes educator, author, Lee walks in your shoes every day. He writes from both clinical and personal experience with honesty, compassion, and humor. He works full time running the diabetes program for a rural nonprofit clinic in one of the poorest counties in the United States, and is a tireless advocate for diabetes care and awareness.

He manages a staff of 8, and has pioneered the *Diabetes Peer Educator* model, using volunteer diabetics to help other patients in ongoing free diabetes education programs. He is the author of the long-running internet blog ***LifeAfterDx*** which chronicles his experiences with the early continuous glucose monitoring technology, his thoughts on diabetes and health politics, and his daily life living with diabetes.

He jokes that he wants his tombstone to read: *Loving husband, devoted father, artist, educator, author. Type-1 Diabetic.* Yes, he wants diabetes on his tombstone so that his great-great-grandchildren can read it and say, "Wow. Poor great-great-grandpa. He actually had to *live* with diabetes. I'm sure glad they cured it."

Other books coming from the pen of William "Lee" Dubois

Coming soon is Lee's long-awaited revolutionary new handbook: ***Real Time Revolution: The art and science of controlling diabetic blood sugar using Continuous Monitoring Systems*** which covers virtually every aspect of continuous monitoring from the technology to the psychology. Widely considered to be the "Godfather" of Continuous Glucose Monitoring, Lee was the 30th person in the United States to get "hooked up" to a CGM system, and may have been using the systems continuously longer than anyone else.

Lee is also penning two other books in his diabetes series: ***So You Love a Diabetic: The complete guide to the care and feeding of your diabetic loved ones***, a handbook for your non-diabetic friends and family to teach them what to do to help you be healthy. Perhaps more importantly, it will teach them what *not* to do, too.

Of course, working as a diabetes educator, Lee is keenly aware that over 4,000 Americans join our ranks every day. He'd love to believe that most of these new members of our "tribe" are getting good advice and good care, but there is plenty of evidence that this is just not the case. So he is writing a handbook for the newly diagnosed entitled: ***Diabetes?! I Can't Possibly Have Diabetes! The handbook for the newly diagnosed diabetic.***